The Health Status of Internal Migrants in China

Peigang Wang
Editor

The Health Status of Internal Migrants in China

Springer

Editor
Peigang Wang
Population and Health Research Center
School of Health Sciences
Wuhan University
Wuhan, China

ISBN 978-981-15-4414-9 ISBN 978-981-15-4415-6 (eBook)
https://doi.org/10.1007/978-981-15-4415-6

This Springer imprint is published by the registered company Springer Nature Singapore Pte Ltd.
The registered company address is: 152 Beach Road, #21-01/04 Gateway East, Singapore 189721, Singapore

Preface

At present, China is in a critical period of socio-economic developmental transformation. The rapid progression of urbanization has absorbed a large number of rural laborers into cities, which contributes to the unprecedented population migration. "China Statistical Yearbook 2019" states that the size of China's internal migrants in 2018 was 241 million people (National Bureau of Statistics, 2020). The large size of the internal migrants has made great contributions to China's social and economic development, but it is not without an owing consequence to the health of migrants. The internal migrants are mainly engaged in labor-intensive work in the inflow areas, with low occupational status, high work intensity, and long working hours. The poor working environment exposes workers to health risks such as dust, noise, and toxic substances, which may lead to occupational diseases such as silicosis, chronic poisoning, and various types of work injuries (Li et al., 2018; Niu, 2013). Weak economic foundation makes it difficult for internal migrants to access high-quality health services or obtain a decent living setting which aggravates their risks for common respiratory and gastrointestinal infectious diseases (Fan, 2019). Urbanization dynamics including work pressure and social isolation also task the mental health of internal migrants (Fan, 2019; Liu, 2018).

In the era of large population movements, population mobility deserves utter attention. For example, the COVID-19 outbreak in China might have accelerated due to the large-scale population movement during the Spring Festival. The high mobility of the internal migrants, the difficulty of tracking and management, and the poor urban living conditions coupled with the weak links in prevention and control further precipitated the endemicity of the outbreak. At present, China's large-scale migration and urbanization of the internal migrants have strained the modernization of urban governance and the modernization of migrant population management services. Solving the health problem of the internal migrants is an integral part of the government's promotion of modernization of social governance. In 2014, the Chinese government launched a pilot project with the aim of equalizing and improving the quality and efficiency of basic public health services for migrants (Yue et al., 2014). The *Outline of "Healthy China 2030" Plan* promulgated in 2019 specifically emphasized the need to address the health issues of the internal migrants when it puts forward the strategic status of people's health as a priority. In addition, health interventions and policies such as medical treatment and reimbursements have continuously been introduced and implemented in various settings, to reduce institutional barriers between the internal migrants and health services. Solving the health problems of the internal migrants does not only help achieve the goals of "*Healthy China*" and "*Health for All*", but is also an inherent requirement for maintaining a healthy society and a stable economy.

All the papers collected in this book are original studies, and they are analyzed using data from the China Migrants Dynamic Survey (2013–2018). As the survey does not provide data on "children and family planning services" in the national database, the team fetched respective content from the 2013–2018 Hubei Provincial Health and Health Committee database. The above data is an annual large-scale national sampling survey of migrants since 2009, covering 31 provinces (autonomous regions and municipalities). The influx of migrants in the Xinjiang Production and Construction Corps is relatively concentrated, with a sample size of nearly 200,000 households per year. It covers basic information on the migrant population and family members including the scope and trend of migration, employment and social security, income and expenditure, and residence, and basic public health services, management of marital and family planning services, child mobility and education, psychological culture, etc. In addition, some years also include the special survey on social integration and mental health of the internal migrants, the special survey on health and family planning services in the outflow areas, and the special survey on medical and health services for the mobile elderly (http://www.chinaldrk.org.cn/wjw/#/home).

This book comprehensively applies cutting-edge research design and analysis methods, integrates trend analysis and causal inference analysis, and considers the potential role of social determinants of health of migrants to provide empirical evidence for scientific interventions. The unique advantage of the internal migrants in the study of the relationship between social factors and health is that it has undergone a huge change in the living environment and the social relationships that have changed with it. Based on this and a dynamic research approach, it is easier to observe significant changes in social factors and health outcomes, which helps to identify the causal relationship between the two and propose targeted interventions.

In an academic sense, this project is at the forefront. It integrates relevant theories and methods, explores the potential causal mechanism in the relationship between social factors and the health of the internal migrants based on the Chinese cultural contexts, which enriches the logical framework of causality between the two. From a practical perspective, in the context of the rapid urbanization and the large size of the internal migrants, solving the health problems of the internal migrants is of a great significance for maintaining the stable development of urban and rural areas, achieving the "*Healthy China 2030*" and the "*Health for All*" goals. General Secretary, Xi Jinping, pointed out that it is necessary to strive to provide quality and comprehensive health services for people throughout their life-course (http://www.xinhuanet.com/health/zt/2016JK20/). Moreover, the *Outline of "Healthy China 2030" Plan* has repeatedly emphasized that a solution must be sought for the health problems of the internal migrants. The current pandemic of COVID-19 also proves that the health problem related to population mobility is a concerning public health issue. Therefore, analyzing and researching the health problems of the internal migrants is not only relevant to the realization of the "*Healthy China 2030*" Goal, but also helps to promote the modernization of the capacity of the national governance system and maintain a healthy socio-economic development of the country.

Wuhan, China Peigang Wang

References

National Bureau of Statistics: China Statistical Yearbook 2019, 2020, China Statistics Press.

Li, J., Wang, T., Sun, Z. (2018). From health advantage to health disadvantage "Epidemiology Paradox" in rural and urban floating population. Population Research, 42(6), 46–60.

Niu, J. (2013). The impact of population mobility on the health differences between urban and rural residents in China, Chinese Social Sciences, (2), 46–63.

Fan, X. (2019). The health status, problems and countermeasures of floating population, Macroeconomic Management, (4), 42–47.

Liu, H. (2018). Actively responding to the mental health problems of the floating population, China Population News (3rd ed.), November 26.

Yue, J., Li, X. (2014). Migrants' health consciousness and utilization of health services from a community perspective: A study based on the pearl river delta, Journal of Public Management, 11(4), 125–135.

http://www.chinaldrk.org.cn/wjw/#/home.

http://www.xinhuanet.com/health/zt/2016JK20/.

Contents

Chapter 1
Migration, Migrants and Health in Flux

Junfeng Jiang

At the time of writing this book, there are more than 240 million internal migrants in flux in China, which is a large number in any country or region. In the setting of social transition, most migrants move from rural to urban areas and become migrant workers or businessmen in China. Migrant workers are products of urbanization and industrialization, and they have made indelible contributions to China's social and economic development. Since most migrants become workers, they need to participate in local labor markets, so health human capital is necessary for the internal migrants in China. Numerous studies observe that, as a kind of human capital, health can largely contribute to socioeconomic development (Grossman, 1972). A better health status can help workers improve their market competitiveness, increase their time available for work, income and opportunities for promotion, and reduce their probability of unemployment (Cheng, Jin, Gai, & Shi, 2014; Ecob & Smith, 1999; Zhang, 2011).

However, plenty of evidence shows that migrants are usually exposed to amounts of health risk factors, including a lower socioeconomic status (SES) (less income, less education, low occupational status), high work intensity or more pressure, social isolation and discrimination, adverse access to health related resources, low-level social integration and adaption (Li, Wang, & Sun, 2018; Niu, 2013). All these risk factors are closely related to series of structural factors, e.g. the household registration system (Wang & Fan, 2012). According to the "healthy migrant effect" theory, although the selection of migration results in a better health status for migrants at the initial stage of migration, these health risk factors will ceaselessly damage migrants' health and lead to a higher health loss rate than average (Chen, 2011; Lu & Qin, 2014; Tong & Piotrowski, 2012). With the deterioration of health condition, the social competitiveness of migrants weakens, forcing them to return to their hometown.

J. Jiang (✉)
School of Health Sciences, Wuhan University, Wuhan, China
e-mail: jiang0111@whu.edu.cn

P. Wang (ed.), *The Health Status of Internal Migrants in China*,
https://doi.org/10.1007/978-981-15-4415-6_1

This health selection effect is called the "salmon bias" (Qi, Niu, Mason, & Treiman, 2012; Ullmann, Goldman, & Massey, 2011). The above two health selections run through the whole process of migration, reflecting the complete process of health change in migrants. Just as the title of this chapter stresses, migrants are in flux, and their health status is also in flux because of their migration.

Migrants' health is a research hotspot in sociology, public health, demography, psychology, economics and many other disciplines in recent years, and over one thousand related studies will be published per year around the world. However, different subjects focus on different aspects of migrants' health. Sociology and demography emphasize the general physical and mental health of migrants and their social determinants; public health or epidemiology emphasizes the mechanism of occurrence and development of various diseases (mainly physiological and pathological mechanisms) and the utilization of health services; psychology emphasizes the relationship between mental health and other factors such as personality and environmental pressure; economics focuses more on the economic causes and forming paths of health, macro-system and health resource distribution, and economic benefits brought by health human capital. It is observed that different subjects have their own advantages in health studies. Medical science focuses more on the refinement of health outcomes and research on various diseases. Although the research on health outcomes in social sciences is not as detailed as that in medical science, the former has more advantages in research methods, emphasizing and applying causal inference methods to find out whether the so-called influencing factors are "real causes" of health. The good news is that many studies on migrants' health present an interdisciplinary characteristic (Qi et al., 2012), which is conducive to a comprehensive understanding of migrants' health. The authors of the following chapters of this book come from sociology, public health, economics and other disciplines, which helps to discuss the health problems of Chinese internal migrants from multiple perspectives.

1 Who Belongs to Migrants?

All of the studies on migrants must define who belongs to migrants, but the concept of migrant has not reached an agreement yet. In China, migration is closely related to the household registration system, the latter stipulates which region an individual belongs to from the perspective of system or law, and accordingly enjoys the responsibilities and obligations within a particular region. Thus, migrants in China are usually internal migrants. Some researchers propose that internal migrants are those who leave their hometown (household registration location) and stay in another place to engage in various economic or other activities (He, 2009). Some researchers stress the characteristic of temporal migration in Chinese internal migrants; that is to say, although they leave their hometown for other places, their household registration usually does not change (Xiong, 2009). Other researchers propose that the characteristic of temporality also requires migrants to return to their permanent residence within a certain period of time (Wang & Hu, 1996; Zhang, 1988). For the time interval of temporality, some researchers propose that people who leave the place of household registration more than half a year can be considered as migrants (Zhai & Duan, 2006), others think there is no need to additionally use time interval to define migrants (Wu & Wang, 2002).

In summary, "unchanged household registration", "leaving household registration location" and "living elsewhere for more than a certain amount of time" are recognized as three main characteristics of migrants by most researchers. In the following chapters of this book, the definition proposed by the National Health Commission of the People's Republic of China is used. That is to say, internal migrants are those who leave their household registration location for other places that belong to another county/district for no less than one month and do not move their household registration to the places they move in. This definition is also in line with the definition widely used in academic researches.

2 Health Status of Internal Migrants in China, also Introducing the "Healthy Migrant Effect" and "Salmon Bias"

In the study on migrants' health, the "healthy migrant effect" and "salmon bias" are two unique health phenomena (Lu & Qin, 2014; Qi et al., 2012). The "healthy migrant effect" (Li et al., 2018) indicates that, at the beginning of moving to other places, migrants are healthier than the natives in the places either they leave or they leave for, which is considered a health selection. However, with the passage of time, migrants' health will gradually deteriorate and usually become poorer than the natives, which is called the "epidemiological paradox" (Chen, 2011; Lu & Qin, 2014). Discussing the social determinants of health during this process is the hot research area in current studies, so most studies on migrants' health focus on the social determinants of health. After the outflow for a period of time, an inevitable choice for migrants is to continue the migration or return home. Evidence shows that there is also a health selection in the backflow of migrants; health status is an important influencing factor of backflow, and migrants who have a poorer health status are more likely to return home (Palloni & Arias, 2004; Qi et al., 2012; Ullmann et al., 2011). This phenomenon is called the "salmon bias". The "healthy migrant effect" and "salmon bias" link the beginning and end of migration, reflecting the whole process of migrants' health change. Studies on the health of international migrants suggest that, after the above two health selections, migrants usually have more advantages in health than the natives (Nauman, VanLandingham, Anglewicz, Patthavanit, & Punpuing, 2015; Palloni & Arias, 2004). In China, however, internal migrants are restrained by multiple institutional and structural factors in the process of migration. Thus, migration brings more health risk factors rather than health protective factors (Li et al., 2018), which leads to more health losses in the process of migration. The health loss and health selection coexist in the process of migration, and there is still no consensus on which one is stronger (Niu, 2013; Shang, Ding, & Shi, 2019; Wang & Zhou, 2018). Therefore, numerous health risk factors are eroding the health of Chinese internal migrants, making their health condition seriously deteriorated, until they return home with a "sick body".

The health problems of Chinese internal migrants are highly related to their low SES and many other social factors. Previous studies indicate that Chinese internal migrants are mainly engaged in labor-intensive work, such as manufacturing, textile and food processing industries, these jobs have the characteristic of low occupational status, high working intensity, long working hours and poor working conditions, and workers in these occupations are more likely to expose to dust, noise, toxic substance and many other health risks. Thus, occupational diseases such as silicosis and chronic intoxication, as well as various occupational injuries, are more common in Chinese internal migrants (Jiang, 2006; Niu, 2013; Zheng & Lian, 2006), and fewer high-quality health resources are available because of their low SES. Also, the low SES of Chinese internal migrants cannot provide them a good living condition, so millions of internal migrants are living in crowded, unfurnished and unsanitary temporal dwellings, and are under the threat of enteritis, tuberculosis and other infectious diseases (Fan, 2019; Zheng & Lian, 2006). Furthermore, as internal migrants are mostly in the stage of frequent reproductive activities, their reproductive health problems are also very serious, and AIDs, abortion, reproductive tract infection and others seriously threaten their health (Zheng & Lian, 2006). Apart from physical health, migrants' psychological health problems are also increasingly severe. For Chinese internal migrants, the incidence of common psychological diseases such as depression is higher than the average level in the entire population, which is closely related to the stress, discrimination and social isolation that they face in the strange land (Fan, 2019). Migrants need to start their new life in an unfamiliar environment, so it is easy for them to have psychological health problems due to social maladjustment, institutional and cultural isolations (Liu, 2018). In the next section, multiple health influencing factors mentioned in other related studies will be systematically summarized and reviewed.

Since many internal migrants are suffering from series of health risks, the Chinese central government takes their health seriously. Since 2009, the Chinese central government has taken up the equalization of basic public health services program, which aims to provide basic public health services for free for all Chinese residents including migrants (Yin et al., 2015). In 2014, the Chinese central government began to carry out the basic public health services program specifically for migrants, which aims to promote the quality and efficiency of the utilization of basic public health services in this special group (Yue & Li, 2014). In addition, medical and health policies such as long-distance medical treatment and reimbursement have also been published and implemented continuously, which has reduced the health system barriers in access to health resources for internal migrants (Ministry of Human Resources and Social Security of China, 2016). Furthermore, the household registration system reform is also gradually reducing the household registration distinction between urban and rural residents, replacing agricultural and non-agricultural household registration with resident household registration, so as to reduce the household registration discrimination of natives on migrants and improve migrants' health. Nevertheless, the health of Chinese internal migrants still faces numerous challenges, and there is still a long way to go for the health for all.

3 Influencing Factors of Migrants' Health

This book mainly focuses on the social determinants of health in Chinese internal migrants, so some socio-demographic factors such as sex and age that may influence migrants' health are not reviewed in this chapter. In this chapter, the health effects of migration factors, SES, social capital, social cohesion and utilization of health services in migrants are reviewed. It should be noted that when examining and discussing the health effect of these factors, readers should not disentangle the internal associations among them and separately analyze them. Instead, readers should understand the health effects of these social determinants from a comprehensive and connected perspective.

3.1 Migration Factors

Migration is a unique characteristic of migrants, and migration factors that may be related to health include range/distance of migration, duration of migration and size of migration. Previous studies observe that a longer distance of migration may have a negative effect on migrants' health; interprovincial migration leads to a decrease in health, while migration within province is not related to health (Qin, Wang, & Jiang, 2014). A longer distance of migration usually yields more cultural and institutional barriers, which may lead to more social maladjustment and less access to health resources and make migrants' health deteriorate. The health effect of duration of migration follows the "healthy migrant effect" and "epidemiological paradox". That is to say, migrants who have a shorter time of migration have a better health status; as time goes by, the health status of migrants will become poorer and even become poorer than the natives. This is closely related to the health risk factors faced by internal migrants in the process of migration, including low-level SES, cultural barriers, social isolation and inconvenient access to health resources (Li et al., 2018; Lu & Qin, 2014). The size of migration mainly refers to family migration, which is also one of the most important trends for Chinese internal migrants. Theoretically speaking, family migration can increase companionship among family members, reduce family tension and increase residential and occupational stability (Taylor & Foster, 2015; Tian, 2014), so as to benefit health. However, although family migration has been observed to be closely related to the social cohesion of migrants (Tian, 2014; Wang & Zhang, 2017), empirical evidence on the causal association between family migration and health is limited.

Based on the review above, it is observed that, in most cases, migration factors are just related to (not causally related to) migrants' health. The association between migration factors and migrants' health exists mainly because these migration factors are associated with series of health risk exposures. Migration factors mentioned above are usually associated with SES, social capital, social cohesion and health services utilization, which are considered to have more important effects on health.

3.2 SES

SES, usually including education, income and occupational status, fundamentally influences health through three ways mainly: improvement of work/living conditions, easy access to health resources, and more health consciousness and health behaviors (Adler & Newman, 2002). The internal migrants in China leave their hometown mainly to find jobs and earn more money, so they have a stronger motivation to pursue high SES, especially high-level income. Thus, SES may have a stronger health effect in Chinese internal migrants. Chinese internal migrants mainly migrate from rural to urban areas, and many disadvantages, including less education, fewer labor skills, less income, high-intensity work, more exposures to health risks and less return on labor, are encountered by them (Chen, Chen, & Landry, 2013; Xie, 2012; Yu & Sun, 2017; Zhao, 2015). Most of the internal migrants, therefore, suffer from a low SES.

For Chinese internal migrants, the health effect of SES still plays a role through the above three ways. Previous evidence shows that poor work conditions, intensive work and less return from work are more likely to be experienced by migrant workers. A continuous exposure to these toxic conditions has led to serious physical wear and more stress in their daily life, which causes a poorer health status of migrants (Chen et al., 2013; Niu, Zheng, Zhang, & Zeng, 2011; Yu, 2016). Furthermore, Chinese internal migrants are mainly rural-to-urban migrants, they usually have a lower level of education that impedes their upward mobility in terms of income and professional status (Jerrim & Macmillan, 2015). Also, their low-level education is not conducive to their social cohesion in values and behaviors and easy to yield social isolation (Hu & Chen, 2012). Furthermore, it is adverse to the access to health information, the development of health consciousness and habits, and the utilization of health resources (Lu, Qiu, Yang, & Qian, 2018). Less education and the shortage of job skills lead to a low occupational status and less income in Chinese internal migrants, and these disadvantages make them unable to obtain high-quality living conditions. This low SES brings numerous health risks, including poor living conditions, less access to health resources, social isolation and exclusion, and a long-term exposure to these risks will inevitably lead to a poor health status for the internal migrants in China (Hu & Chen, 2012; Li et al., 2018; Liang, Hou, & Li, 2017; Niu, 2013; Yu & Zhu, 2018).

3.3 Social Capital and Social Cohesion

Social capital and social cohesion are two important social determinants of health, and they have not only some distinctions but some overlaps. Social capital usually refers to social resources, norms of reciprocity and trust produced by and nested in the social connections across social members, so trust, norms of reciprocity, social interaction and participation are widely used to measure social capital (Putnam, 2001, 2002). By contrast, social cohesion usually refers to the integration in economy, culture/values, social network and identity after migrants migrate into a new place (Chen & Zhang, 2015; Yang, 2015; Zhou, 2012). It can be observed that the two concepts overlap in social participation, social network and interactions: the active participation in local social activities and interactions with the natives are common ways to improve social capital and social cohesion, and they are also frequently-used measures of these two things.

Since the concept and measure of social capital and social cohesion are complex, current empirical evidence on the relationship between social capital/social cohesion and health is mixed. Studies on social capital and health in migrants are still rare, and most of them observe a positive association between social capital and health. For example, trust and social participation are observed to be two important protective factors of health for migrants in Sweden (Lecerof, Stafström, Westerling, & Östergren, 2016); family network can improve the psychological health of migrants by increasing the social support obtained from their family members in Indonesia (Lu, 2012); and various forms of social participation, including bonding, bridging and linking, can improve the self-rated health (SRH) of migrants by reducing discriminations from others in Korea (Kim, 2016). Although social capital is observed to have a positive effect on the physical and mental health of Chinese internal migrants (Wang & Chen, 2015), more evidence suggests that different forms of social capital have distinct effects on migrants' health (Hu & Chen, 2012; Palmer & Xu, 2013). For example, Hu and Chen (2012) proposed that more trust and intensive social networks were related to better psychological health in Chinese internal migrants, but a higher level of heterogeneity in networks reduced their psychological health, as heterogeneous networks increased discrimination and social pressure. Palmer and Xu (2013) observed that individual-focused social capital (friend and family support), trust in community members and community attachment had positive health effects in Chinese rural-to-urban migrants, but neighboring and organizational social capital had negative health effects. Using the instrumental variable approach, Mi, Li, and Zhu (2016) observed that the positive health effect of social network was stronger than of trust and norms of reciprocity in Chinese internal migrants, and their social connection to the natives brought more health benefits than to the people in their hometown. Other researches indicate that social capital can improve health by reducing the exposure to series of health risks (Qiaohong Yang, Zaller, Huang, Dong, & Zhang, 2018; Yang, Li, & Attane, 2015).

More studies on social cohesion and health are published. Studies in different cultural settings suggest that social cohesion usually has a positive effect on the physical and psychological health of migrants (Hong, Zhang, & Walton, 2014; Ruijsbroek, Droomers, Hardyns, Groenewegen, & Stronks, 2016; Vries, Dillen, Groenewegen, & Spreeuwenberg, 2013; Wang & Chen, 2015). Furthermore, social cohesion is considered a multidimensional concept, and each dimension is closely related to health. Evidence from European countries suggests that elevated country-level social cohesion is related to better SRH in migrants (Chuang, Chuang, & Yang, 2013; Deindl, Brandt, & Hank, 2016). And micro-level evidence suggests that migrants' health is closely related to their employment status, level of income and working conditions (Berkman, Kawachi, & Glymour, 2014), which implies the importance of economic cohesion for migrant workers' health. Migrants' integration in local social networks and participation in local social activities can also improve their physical health. A higher level of social participation, including participating in religious activities and neighborhood/community activities, contributes to better physical health (Ikeda & Kawachi, 2010; Muennig, Cohen, Palmer, & Zhu, 2013); and a higher level of peer social networks usually provides more social support and connections, and reduces pressure and hostility, which helps individuals obtain more health resources and improve their health (Link & Phelan, 1995). For psychological health, evidence from developed countries shows that, for migrants, a higher level of cohesion in social network and participation is related to better psychological health (Ikeda & Kawachi, 2010; Muennig et al., 2013), and elevated neighborhood cohesion is associated with reduced depression (Perez et al., 2015) and elevated psychological health (Erdem, Lenthe, Prins, Voorham, & Burdorf, 2016; Erdem, Prins, Voorham, Lenthe, & Burdorf, 2015).

Studies on the mechanism of social cohesion affecting health mainly focus on the role of social cohesion in promoting the health behaviors of migrants (Holmes & Marcelli, 2014; Kim & Kawachi, 2017). Previous evidence shows that a higher level of perceived social cohesion is closely related to a lower probability of excessive drinking (Ma & Smith, 2017). Neighborhood cohesion can help reduce the smoking behaviors of migrants (Holmes & Marcelli, 2014; Lozano et al., 2016) and the probability of smoking among migrants who have children (Alcalá, Sharif, & Albert, 2016). A higher level of perceived neighborhood cohesion also benefits the access to high-quality healthcare resources and services (Kim & Kawachi, 2017; Maleku, Kim, & Lee, 2019). Thus, elevated social cohesion produces better health by increasing health behaviors in most situations in migrant population.

3.4 *Health Resources and Services*

Some studies consider that a higher SES and elevated social capital and cohesion can improve migrants' health by increasing their convenience of access to health resources (Hou, Lin, & Zhang, 2017; Lu et al., 2018; Maleku et al., 2019). It is recognized that the access and utilization of health resources and services are downstream influencing factors of health, which have a direct protective effect on migrants' health, particularly physical health. Previous evidence suggests that an equal access to basic public health services, such as medical insurance intake (Song & Zhang, 2018) and health education engagement (Liu, Gao, & Zhang, 2018), contributes to the promotion of migrants' health, where the most direct way is to increase the access to health resources and the efficiency of health resources utilization (Cai, Yang, & Bian, 2019; Han & Meng, 2019). Although some evidence from developed countries suggests that the utilization of healthcare services in migrants is not less than in local residents (Rodriguez-Alvarez, Lanborena, & Borrell, 2019), a huge disadvantage in the utilization of healthcare services in Chinese internal migrants can be observed because of numerous structural or institutional factors (Shao et al., 2018; Zheng, Hu, Dong, & Hao, 2018). In this unique setting, the central government of China has carried out the plot project of equal access to basic public health services to improve the quality and efficiency of the utilization of basic public health services among migrants (Yue & Li, 2014).

4 Focuses in Empirical Studies: Contextual Factors and Causal Effects

The study design and statistical method have also become more and more detailed, accurate and advanced in recently published studies on migrants' health, specific contexts and unique health problems have also be taken seriously. Thus, two issues have been paid attention to in studies on migrants' health. One is the contextual social determinant of health in migrants, another is the causal health effect of social determinants.

The generalized multilevel model is widely used when it comes to the contextual effect on health. The environment that migrants live in, including the level of infrastructure, working place environment and neighborhood conditions, will have a profound effect on their health behaviors and outcomes (Levecque & Rossem, 2015; Lu & Wang, 2019; Niu et al., 2011), and they are a kind of macro factors that are independent of specific migrants. Actually, individuals sharing the same living environment usually have stronger connections, while individuals sharing distinct living environments usually have some systematic differences. However, the generalized linear model requires the assumption of sample independence, and there should be no systematic difference across different groups. Thus, a biased estimation will be yielded in most situations. By contrast, the generalized multilevel model does not require such assumption and can estimate the contextual effects of macro influencing factors more accurately (Wang, Xie, & Jiang, 2008). In common two-level nested models, the contextual effects of environmental factors in local areas on migrants' health can be examined. Furthermore, in cross-classified random effects models (CCREM), the contextual effects of both local environmental factors and hometown environmental factors on migrants' health can be simultaneously examined. In three—or more-level nested models, researchers can examine the health effects of factors from multi-levels. The multilevel model is used to estimate the contextual effects of group factors on migrants' health in this book. For example, Chap. 10 uses community as the group level and discusses the influence of community factors on female migrants' contraceptive behaviors. Chap. 11 uses province as the group level and examines the health effect of province-level economic development in Chinese internal elderly migrants.

Another important issue is that specific causal inference approaches should be used in empirical studies on migrants' health, as the migration itself is a selection. The health of migrants has a characteristic of selection, and it is obviously reflected in the phenomena of "healthy migrant effect" and "salmon bias". The former indicates a health selection at the beginning of migration, while the latter indicates a health selection at the end of migration. Related studies using a causal inference design can be classified into two categories. One uses longitudinal data, design and methods to observe the health trajectories with time to yield the causal health effect of other factors (Lu & Qin, 2014; Nauman et al., 2015); another uses specific causal inference approaches, such as the instrumental variables (IV), propensity scores matching (PSM) and difference-in-difference (DID) approaches, to yield the causal effect on health (Shang et al., 2019; Wang & Zhou, 2018). This book also focuses on the application of some causal inference designs and approaches when it comes to migrants' health, which is interspersed in some chapters. For example, Chap. 4 discusses and addresses potential endogeneity problems from multiple perspectives to yield a more accurate causal association between minimum wage standard and migrants' social medical insurance take-up. PSM was used to do a robust check in Chaps. 7 and 11 to provide more strong evidence for the association between migration experience and migrants' health, as well as the positive association between the education of migrant children and the health of their older parents.

5 Framework, Contents and Innovations of this Book

There are 11 chapters in this book. This Chapter is an introduction that briefly reviews the concept of migrants, as well as some hot issues and empirical methods widely used in migrants' health studies. The core contents and data used in the following chapters are also introduced in this Chapter. General internal migrants in China are analyzed in Chaps. 2–7, while Chaps. 8–11 discuss some special groups such as female and older migrants.

The status quo and influencing factors of basic public health services among Chinese internal migrants are discussed in Chap. 2. Nationally representative data and data from Hubei Province were used, and the establishment of health record (HR) and receiving of health education (HE) were analyzed. It is reported that the utilization level of HR and HE in migrant population was moderate, migrants with low SES and without medical insurance should be paid more attention to. The equalization of basic public health services is an important policy vigorously promoted by Chinese central government in recent years to improve migrants' health (Yue & Li, 2014).

Therefore, the investigation on the basic public health services of migrants can help find good ways to improve policies as well as their health.

Because migrants' health usually deteriorates with time in local areas, good health seeking behaviors will help maintain their health. However, the choice of health seeking behaviors is a complicated issue for migrants, as it involves the medical treatment and settlement in different places. Most migrants have heavier disease burdens and long to obtain better health resources at less cost. However, the reimbursement ratio of different medical insurance for the treatment of various diseases is different, so the type of medical insurance will influence the medical treatment choice of migrant population. Accordingly, Chap. 3 analyzes the influence of migration direction and range on the health seeking behavior of migrant population. We found that the type of medical insurance indeed affected hospitalization behaviors and medical expense reimbursement ratio in Chinese internal migrants, and these effects were significantly different in migrants with different migration directions. These findings will help to provide some insights into the reform of China's healthcare system.

Chapter 4 investigates the influence of local minimum wage standard on social health insurance in Chinese internal migrants. Migrants usually have less income than the natives, so their income is more likely to be influenced by local minimum wage standard. Because income is an important basis of social health insurance take-up, a higher level of local minimum wage standard may have a stronger protective effect for migrants. However, this chapter found that elevated minimum wage standard could not only increase migrants' social health insurance take-up by increasing their income, but also reduce migrants' social health insurance take-up due to the potential substitution between income and health insurance. This chapter re-examined the causal relationship between minimum wage standard and social health insurance and highlighted the importance of improving the ability of China's current medical insurance programs to obtain high-quality health resources.

Chapters 5 and 6 investigate the influence of social cohesion on migrants' health and life satisfaction. Chapter 5 found that migrants with different identity patterns had different physical and mental health outcomes, while Chap. 6 observed that perceived stress was a mediator in the relationship between economic cohesion/social participation and life satisfaction, and this mediation effect was stronger in migrants with a higher level of identity. The perspective of social cohesion is the most common and relevant one in migrants' health studies, it is also considered one of the cores frameworks in relevant studies (Lu et al., 2018). The deterioration of migrants' health is closely related to the accumulation of pressure and poor social cohesion (Sirin, Gupta, & Rogers-Sirin, 2013). Therefore, the "healthy migrant effect" and "salmon bias" are closely related to the social cohesion of migrants. More attention to the health effect of social cohesion can help explore the theoretical basis of health transformation and related phenomena among Chinese internal migrants.

Issues on the "healthy migrant effect" and "salmon bias" have been widely discussed in prior studies. Thus, Chap. 7 tries to re-examine the effect of migration experiences on the health of Chinese internal migrants. This chapter focuses on the effects of migration duration and number of city that has ever migrated in on migrants' health. Potential selection problem is addressed using PSM approach, and potential group disparities in the above two effects are also examined. The results show that the health of migrants with more education and urban *hukou* is not influenced by migration duration, and the health of migrants with more family income seems not to be influenced by migration experiences. As health selection cannot be ignored when it comes to migrants' health, these results re-confirm the "salmon bias" and enrich the theoretical connotations of health selection theory.

Chapters 8–10 focus on female migrants and discuss some issues on marriage and fertility; Chap. 8 highlights the cohort disparity in marriage and fertility outcomes, Chap. 9 focuses on the first birth interval of female migrants, and Chap. 10 investigates multilevel influencing factors of contraceptive behaviors in female migrants, especially community and policy factors. We found that there were cohort effects on the marriage and fertility of female migrants (e.g., time of marriage, birth interval, and abortion); community-level basic public health services significantly influenced the contraceptive behaviors of migrant females, and there are also substantial impacts of the Two-Child Policy on the contraceptive behaviors of migrant females. The difference in generation/cohort is not only difference in age, but difference in life experiences and living conditions, or called difference in life course. Individuals born in different eras will have huge differences in early life experiences, values, behavior patterns and health awareness, so they may have differences in health behaviors and outcomes (Jiang & Wang, 2018; Jones et al., 2019). Currently, the new generation (post-80s and 90s generations) has gradually become the main force of China's migrant population. Thus, comparing the health-related outcomes and mechanisms between old and new generations can help grasp the transition in health outcomes and the social determinants of health. Female migrants belong to one of the vulnerable groups in migrants, and marriage and fertility issues in female migrants are also focuses in migrants' health studies. The investigation on the influence of cohort and community-level factors can help to generate interventions from a broader perspective, so as to improve the health of migrant females.

The last chapter mainly discusses the influence of migrants' education on their accompanying elderly parents' health. The number of older migrants has increased in recent years, and they usually have a poorer health status and require more health resources (Song & Zhang, 2018). Because older migrants usually migrate with and largely rely on their children, their health is highly related to the economic capability of their children. According to the human resource theory, education is an important reflection of economic ability, so, for migrants, more education can guarantee the acquisition of health resources for their accompanying elderly parents and display a positive externality. Therefore, Chap. 11 tries to discuss the causal relationship between migrants' education and their accompanying elderly parents' health in China. It is reported that there was a robust positive causal association between migrants' education and their accompanying elderly parents' health, and the education difference between migrants and their accompanying elderly parents negatively affected their health. These findings may provide some insights on the promotion of older migrants' health.

This book strives to be innovative in both contents and methods. As mentioned in the introduction above, some detailed and comprehensive analyses on major issues (e.g., Chaps. 2, 6 and 8), as well as in-depth study on some hot issues (e.g., Chaps. 3 and 10) are displayed to reflect the content innovation. In addition, this book introduces some advanced research points into migrants' health study (e.g., intergenerational feeding in Chap. 11) and highlights the frontier and novelty of our research contents.

Taking advantage of multi-disciplinary advantages, we try to introduce multi-disciplinary quantitative methods and emphasize on the principle of detailedness, accuracy and logicality. For example, Chap. 4 adjusts for the regional fixed effect and highlights the principle of accuracy, it also discusses the influence mechanism and population heterogeneity to highlight detailedness and logicality. In Chap. 5, the latent class analysis (LCA) is applied to classify identity in a more accurate way. Chapter 6 combines mediating and moderating effects into the structural equation model (SEM) to reflect the principle of detailedness and logicality. In Chap. 11, an interaction analysis is introduced into multilevel model, and PSM is also used to yield accurate estimations. Using these statistical methods, this book seeks to obtain robust evidence.

6 A Brief Introduction to the Data Source

The data used in all empirical chapters of this book are obtained from the China Migrants Dynamic Survey (CMDS). The CMDS is held by the National Health Commission of the People's Republic of China, it is a cross-sectional survey and has been carried out year by year since 2009. A stratified multi-stage probability-proportional-to-size sampling (PPS) method was used, a total of 31 provincial administrative units were covered, and 160,000–200,000 nationally representative migrants were interviewed in each survey. During 2009–2014, migrants aged from 15 to 59 years old were interviewed; by contrast, migrants aged 15 or older have been interviewed since 2015, which includes older migrants aged 60 or older. In all surveys, migrants were defined as individuals who lived in local areas no less than one month but the household registration location of them did not belong to this district/county/city. It should be noted that the following three groups are not included in CMDS: one of the couple is migrant but another is the native; parents are migrants but children are the natives; soldiers and students.

Although the questionnaires used are not quite the same from year to year, they mainly include the following contents: (1) basic information of migrants and their family members, including sex, age, education, marital status, migration characteristics etc. (2) detailed migration experiences, including duration of migration, people that migrate together, willingness of migration etc. (3) work status and income in local areas; (4) social cohesion, including cohesion in community engagement, living habits, social networks, identity etc. (5) health outcomes and the utilization of public health services, including health seeking behaviors, participation in health insurance etc. In addition to personal information above, the survey also collects some community information, including infrastructure, progress of healthcare and family planning work etc. Therefore, the survey provides a high-quality data support for a comprehensive analysis on the health of Chinese internal migrants.

The CMDS is the most comprehensive national micro survey for Chinese internal migrants, which has obvious advantages in the quality, openness, succession and representation of data. Its characteristic of large sample also conforms to the development of healthy big data. Based on the data from CMDS, numerous studies on the health of Chinese internal migrants have been published in some top journals. Internationally, for example, based on the data collected in 2012, Ji et al. (2016) discussed the status quo and influencing factors of smoking by sex in Chinese internal migrants; they observed that education, social cohesion and other factors reduced the possibility of migrants' smoking behaviors in China. Based on the data collected in 2015, using DID models, Lu, Chen, and Wang (2019) observed that language barriers had a negative effect on older migrants' health in China by hindering their construction of social network. Using the CMDS data of 2014, Wang, Zhang, Hou, Yan, and Hou (2018) observed that medical insurance only had a weak effect on the health seeking behaviors of Chinese internal migrants, so they suggested that the unity of medical insurance should be strengthened to improve the positive influence of medical insurance on health seeking behaviors. By contrast, Peng and Ling (2019) found that migrants' health seeking behaviors after returning home were associated with the place where they purchased their medical insurance, and migrants who purchased their medical insurance in their hometown were more likely to go to see a doctor at home; thus, it was necessary to establish a communication mechanism among interregional medical and health systems.

More related studies using the CMDS data can be found in journals in Chinese. For example, based on the data collected in 2013, Yang (2015) studied the multi-level influencing factors, including individual- and community-level factors, of social cohesion in Chinese internal migrants; she found a low level of social cohesion and large differences in various dimensions of social cohesion and proposed that a good health services environment within communities and the acceptance of the natives were associated with better social cohesion in this special group. Based on the data collected in 2014, Ma, Qu, and Song (2018) discussed potential reasons that caused the inequality of opportunity in access to health resources using PSM-DID models; they concluded that an integrated medical insurance system could partly reduce the gap in access to healthcare resources caused by the household registration system. Based on the data collected in 2015, Yu and Sun (2017) observed that the ever-widening income gap between migrants with urban *hukou* and migrants with rural *hukou* were mainly attributed to the discrimination on *hukou*, which was adverse to the health gain of migrants with rural *hukou*. By contrast, Song and Zhang (2018) concluded that although an obvious health selection made older migrants in China healthier, they still faced numerous health risks, such as low-level medical insurance take-up, less-frequency physical exercise, low SES and other migration factors.

This book tries to discuss the health of Chinese internal migrants deeply and comprehensively, focusing on the social determinants of health and ways to improve the equal distribution and utilization of health resources. These contents are also a reply to the modern medical model of "physiological-psychological-social". A small sign can indicate a great trend. We hope this book can help the readers understand the living condition and health status of Chinese internal migrants, a common and unique group that has appeared and rapidly expanded in the background of rapid social transition, and how the improvement of their health disadvantages is possible. In the process of social transition in the next few decades, internal migrants will still play a key role in the social development of China, and the health status of this unique group will also be paid much attention to for a long time.

References

Adler, N. E., & Newman, K. (2002). Socioeconomic disparities in health: Pathways and policies. *Health Affairs, 21*(2), 60–76.

Alcalá, H. E., Sharif, M. Z., & Albert, S. L. (2016). Social cohesion and the smoking behaviors of adults living with children. *Addictive Behaviors, 53,* 201–205.

Berkman, L. F., Kawachi, I., & Glymour, M. M. (2014). *Social epidemiology*. New York: Oxford University Press.

Cai, X., Yang, F., & Bian, Y. (2019). Gap analysis on hospitalized health service utilization in floating population covered by different medical insurances: Case study from Jiangsu Province, China. *International Journal for Equality in Health, 18,* e84.

Chen, J. (2011). Internal migration and health: Re-examining the healthy migrant phenomenon in China. *Social Science and Medicine, 72*(8), 1294–1301.

Chen, J., Chen, S., & Landry, P. F. (2013). Migration, environmental hazards, and health outcomes in China. *Social Science and Medicine, 80,* 85–95.

Chen, Y., & Zhang, Y. (2015). The inequality effect and social integration in urbanization. *Social Sciences in China* (6), 78–95.

Cheng, M., Jin, Y., Gai, Q. E., & Shi, Q. (2014). Focusing on education or health improvement for anti-poverty in rural China: Evidence from national household panel data. *Economic Research Journal* (11), 130–144.

Chuang, Y.-C., Chuang, K.-Y., & Yang, T.-H. (2013). Social cohesion matters in health. *International Journal for Equality in Health, 12,* e87.

Deindl, C., Brandt, M., & Hank, K. (2016). Social networks, social cohesion, and later-life health. *Social Indicators Research, 126,* 1175–1187.

Ecob, R., & Smith, G. D. (1999). Income and health: What is the nature of the relationship? *Social Science and Medicine, 48*(5), 693–705.

Erdem, Ö., Lenthe, F. J. V., Prins, R. G., Voorham, T. A. J. J., & Burdorf, A. (2016). Socioeconomic inequalities in psychological distress among urban adults: The moderating role of neighborhood social cohesion. *PLoS ONE, 11*(6), e0157119.

Erdem, Ö., Prins, R. G., Voorham, T. A. J. J., Lenthe, F. J. v., & Burdorf, A. (2015). Structural neighbourhood conditions, social cohesion and psychological distress in the Netherlands. *European Journal of Public Health, 25*(6), 995–1001.

Fan, X. (2019). Health status of Chinese migrants: Problems and countermeasures. *Macroeconomic Management* (4), 42–47.

Grossman, M. (1972). On the concept of health capital and the demand for health. *Journal of Political Economy, 80*(2), 223–255.

Han, J., & Meng, Y. (2019). Institutional differences and geographical disparity: The impact of medical insurance on the equality of health services utilization by the floating elderly population: Evidence from China. *International Journal for Equality in Health, 18,* e91.

He, Z. (2009). *The roadmap of social management reform in China*. Beijing: National School of Administration Press.

Holmes, L. M., & Marcelli, E. A. (2014). Neighborhood social cohesion and smoking among legal and unauthorized Brazilian migrants in Metropolitan Boston. *Journal of Urban Health: Bulletin of the New York Academy of Medicine, 91*(6), 1175–1188.

Hong, S., Zhang, W., & Walton, E. (2014). Neighborhoods and mental health: Exploring ethnic density, poverty, and social cohesion among Asian Americans and Latinos. *Social Science and Medicine, 111,* 117–124.

Hou, Z., Lin, S., & Zhang, D. (2017). Social capital, neighbourhood characteristics and utilisation of local public health services among domestic migrants in China: A cross-sectional study. *British Medical Journal Open, 7*(8), e014224.

Hu, R., & Chen, S. (2012). Social factors influencing peasant workers' mental health. *Chinese Journal of Sociology, 32*(6), 135–157.

Ikeda, A., & Kawachi, I. (2010). *Social networks and health*. New York: Oxford University Press.

Jerrim, J., & Macmillan, L. (2015). Income inequality, intergenerational mobility, and the Great Gatsby Curve: Is education the key? *Social Forces, 94*(2), 505–533.

Ji, Y., Liu, S., Zhao, X., Jiang, Y., Zeng, Q., & Chang, C. (2016). Smoking and its determinants in Chinese internal migrants: Nationally representative cross-sectional data analyses. *Nicotine & Tobacco Research, 18*(8), 1719–1726.

Jiang, C. (2006). Pressure on health burden of migrant workers in unfair employment environment and its alleviation. *Reform of Economic System* (5), 111–114.

Jiang, J., & Wang, P. (2018). Health status in a transitional society: Urban-rural disparities from a dynamic perspective in China. *Population Health Metrics, 16,* e22.

Jones, N. L., Gilman, S. E., Cheng, T. L., Drury, S. S., Hill, C. V., & Geronimus, A. T. (2019). Life course approaches to the causes of health disparities. *American Journal of Public Health, 109*(S1), S48–S55.

Kim, C.-O. (2016). Discrimination-related health inequality and role of social capital among marriage migrant women in South Korea. *International Journal for Equity in Health, 15,* e176.

Kim, E. S., & Kawachi, I. (2017). Perceived neighborhood social cohesion and preventive healthcare use. *American Journal of Preventive Medicine, 53*(2), 35–40.

Lecerof, S. S., Stafström, M., Westerling, R., & Östergren, P.-O. (2016). Does social capital protect mental health among migrants in Sweden? *Health Promotion International, 31*(3), 644–652.

Levecque, K., & Rossem, R. V. (2015). Depression in Europe: Does migrant integration have mental health payoffs? A cross-national comparison of 20 European countries. *Ethnicity & Health, 20*(1), 49–65.

Li, J., Wang, T., & Sun, Z. (2018). From health advantage to health disadvantage: The epidemiological paradox in rural migrants. *Population Research, 42*(6), 46–60.

Liang, Y., Hou, B., & Li, S. (2017). The influence of living pressure and living conditions on the mental health of migrant workers. *Urban Problems* (9), 94–103.

Link, B. G., & Phelan, J. (1995). Social conditions as fundamental causes of disease. *Journal of Health & Social Behavior, Extra Issue: Forty Years of Medical Sociology: The State of the Art and Directions for the Future, 35,* S80–S94.

Liu, H. (2018). Dealing with the mental health problems of migrants actively, *China Population News*.

Liu, L., Gao, H., & Zhang, Y. (2018). The psychological health of floating population and its determinants: The perspective of community integration. *Fudan Journal (Social Sciences Edition)* (4), 158–166.

Lozano, P., Fleischer, N. L., Moore, S., Shigematsu, L. M. R., Santillá, E. A., & Thrasher, J. F. (2016). Does neighborhood social cohesion modify the relationship between neighborhood social norms and smoking behaviors in Mexico? *Health & Place, 40,* 145–152.

Lu, H., Qiu, H., Yang, L., & Qian, W. (2018). Review and analytical framework on rural-urban migrants' health research. *Issues in Agricultural Economy* (1), 110–120.

Lu, N., & Wang, Y. (2019). Neighborhood and mental health of migrants in China. *Journal of Social Development, 6*(2), 175–189.

Lu, S., Chen, S., & Wang, P. (2019). Language barriers and health status of elderly migrants: Micro-evidence from China. *China Econimic Review, 54*, 94–112.

Lu, Y. (2012). Household migration, social support, and psychosocial health: The perspective from migrant-sending areas. *Social Science and Medicine, 74*(2), 135–142.

Lu, Y., & Qin, L. (2014). Healthy migrant and salmon bias hypotheses: A study of health and internal migration in China. *Social Science and Medicine, 102*, 41–48.

Ma, C., Qu, Z., & Song, Z. (2018). Inequality of opportunity of floating population' health care under the integrated medical insurance system: Paradox of the ex-ante or ex-post compensation principle. *China Industrial Economics* (2), 100–117.

Ma, C., & Smith, T. E. (2017). Increased alcohol use after Hurricane Ike: The roles of perceived social cohesion and social control. *Social Science and Medicine, 190*, 29–37.

Maleku, A., Kim, Y. K., & Lee, G. (2019). Social cohesion and immigrant health: Does language-efficacy matter? *International Journal of Migration, Health and Social Care, 15*(1), 17–30.

Ministry of Human Resources and Social Security of China. (2016). Notice of direct settlement of medical expenses for basic medical insurance across provinces. Retrieved from http://www.mohrss.gov.cn/gkml/zcfg/gfxwj/201612/t20161215_262040.html.

Mi, S., Li, B., & Zhu, Q. (2016). The impact of social captial on the health status of rural-urban migrant workers. *Issues in Agricultural Economy, 37*(9), 42–53.

Muennig, P., Cohen, A. K., Palmer, A., & Zhu, W. (2013). The relationship between five different measures of structural social capital, medical examination outcomes, and mortality. *Social Science and Medicine, 85*(3), 18–26.

Nauman, E., VanLandingham, M., Anglewicz, P., Patthavanit, U., & Punpuing, S. (2015). Rural-to-urban migration and changes in health among young adults in Thailand. *Demography, 52*(1), 233–257.

Niu, J. (2013). Migration and its impact on the differences in health between rural and urban residents in China. *Social Sciences in China* (2), 46–63.

Niu, J., Zheng, Z., Zhang, L., & Zeng, X. (2011). Labor migrants' working and living environments and the related health impacts: Evidence from Shenzhen. *Population Research, 35*(3), 64–75.

Palloni, A., & Arias, E. (2004). Paradox lost: Explaining the hispanic adult mortality advantage. *Demography, 41*(3), 385–415.

Palmer, N., & Xu, Q. (2013). Social capital, migration and health in the urban Chinese context. *Journal of Ethnic and Migration Studies, 39*(1), 31–50.

Peng, B.-L., & Ling, L. (2019). Association between rural-to-urban migrants' social medical insurance, social integration and their medical return in China: A national representative cross-sectional data analysis. *BMC Public Health, 19*, e86.

Perez, L. G., Arredondo, E. M., McKenzie, T. L., Holguin, M., Elder, J. P., & Ayala, G. X. (2015). Neighborhood social cohesion and depressive symptoms among Latinos: Does use of community resources for physical activity matter? *Journal of Physical Activity & Health, 12*(10), 1361–1368.

Putnam, R. D. (2001). Social capital: Measurement and consequences. *Canadian Journal of Policy Research, 2*(1), 41–51.

Putnam, R. D. (2002). *Democracies in flux: The evolution of social capital in contemporary society*. New York: Oxford University Press.

Qi, Y., Niu, J., Mason, W., & Treiman, D. (2012). China's internal migration and health selection effect. *Population Research, 36*(1), 102–112.

Qiaohong Yang, D. O., Zaller, N., Huang, W., Dong, Y., & Zhang, H. (2018). Depression and its correlations with health risk behaviors and social capital among female migrants working in entertainment venues in China. *PLoS ONE, 13*(2), e0191632.

Qin, L., Wang, Z., & Jiang, Z. (2014). The migration and health of migrant workers in China: Panel evidence based on relocation sites. *World Economic Papers* (6), 44–59.

Rodriguez-Alvarez, E., Lanborena, N., & Borrell, L. N. (2019). Health services access inequalities between native and immigrant in a southern European region. *International Journal of Health Services, 49*(1), 108–126.

Ruijsbroek, A., Droomers, M., Hardyns, W., Groenewegen, P. P., & Stronks, K. (2016). The interplay between neighbourhood characteristics: the health impact of changes in social cohesion, disorder and unsafety feelings. *Health & Place, 39,* 1–8.

Shang, Y., Ding, S., & Shi, Z. (2019). The health selection or the migration effects? An analysis of the health differentials between different migration type of the rural labor. *South China Population, 34*(3), 13–24.

Shao, S., Wang, M., Jin, G., Zhao, Y., Lu, X., & Du, J. (2018). Analysis of health service utilization of migrants in Beijing using Anderson health service utilization model. *BMC Health Services Research, 18,* e462.

Sirin, S. R., Gupta, T., & Rogers-Sirin, L. (2013). The role of acculturative stress on mental health symptoms for immigrant adolescents: A longitudinal investigation. *Development Psychology, 49*(4), 736–748.

Song, Q., & Zhang, Q. (2018). Research on health status of the elderly migrant population in China and its determinants. *Chinese Journal of Population Science* (4), 81–92.

Taylor, A., & Foster, J. (2015). Migrant workers and the problem of social cohesion in Canada. *Journal of International Migration and Integration, 16*(1), 153–172.

Tian, Y. (2014). Comparison of urban assimilation between family and non-family rural migrants. *Issues in Agricultural Economy*(12), 53–62.

Tong, Y., & Piotrowski, M. (2012). Migration and health selectivity in the context of internal migration in China, 1997-2009. *Population Research and Policy Review, 31*(4), 497–543.

Ullmann, S. H., Goldman, N., & Massey, D. S. (2011). Healthier before they migrate, less healthy when they return? The health of returned migrants in Mexico. *Social Science and Medicine, 73*(3), 421–428.

Vries, S. d., Dillen, S. M. E. v., Groenewegen, P. P., & Spreeuwenberg, P. (2013). Streetscape greenery and health: stress, social cohesion and physical activity as mediators. *Social Science & Medicine, 94*, 26–33.

Wang, C., & Zhang, C. (2017). Migrant children and rural-urban migrant's integration to the city. *Sociological Research* (2), 199–224.

Wang, H., Zhang, D., Hou, Z., Yan, F., & Hou, Z. (2018). Association between social health insurance and choice of hospitals among internal migrants in China: A national cross-sectional study. *British Medical Journal Open, 8,* e018440.

Wang, J., & Hu, Q. (1996). *Chinese internal migrants*. Shanghai: Shanghai University of Finance & Economics Press.

Wang, J., Xie, H., & Jiang, B. (2008). *Multilevel methods and application*. Beijing: Higher Education Press.

Wang, L., & Zhou, H. (2018). Migration and health selectivity. *Northwest Population, 39*(6), 13–22.

Wang, P., & Chen, X. (2015). Social capital, social cohesion and health attainment: Taking example for rural-to-urban migrants. *Journal of Huazhong University of Science and Technology (Social Science Edition), 29*(3), 81–88.

Wang, W. W., & Fan, C. C. (2012). Migrant workers' integration in urban China: Experiences in employment, social adaptation, and self-identity. *Eurasian Geography and Economics, 53*(6), 731–749.

Wu, W., & Wang, H. (2002). Living in big cities: The housing conditions of migrants in Beijing and Shanghai. *Sociological Research* (3), 92–110.

Xie, G. (2012). Returns to human capital and social integration of migrants in China. *Social Sciences in China* (4), 103–124.

Xiong, G. (2009). *Research on the political exclusion of Chinese migrants*. Beijing: China Renmin University Press.

Yang, B., Li, S., & Attane, I. (2015). Risky sexual behaviors among male migrants: Perspective of socioeconomic status and social capital. *Nanjing Journal of Social Sciences* (1), 91–99.

Yang, J. (2015). Research on the assimilation of the floating population in China. *Social Sciences in China* (2), 61–79.

Yin, D., Wong, S. T., Chen, W., Xin, Q., Wang, L., Cui, M., et al. (2015). A model to estimate the cost of the National Essential Public Health Services Package in Beijing, China. *BMC Public Health, 15,* e222.

Yu, L. (2016). The effects of living conditions and working environment on health to the new generation migrant workers. *Zhejiang Social Sciences* (5), 75–84.

Yu, L., & Zhu, Y. (2018). The influence of residential segregation on migrants' health: Based on the national dynamic monitoring of migrant health survey in 2014. *Shandong Social Sciences* (6), 120–128.

Yu, X., & Sun, Y. (2017). The income difference between rural and urban floating migrants: The quantile regression based on data of 2015 dynamic monitoring of floating population. *Population Research, 41*(1), 84–97.

Yue, J., & Li, X. (2014). Health consciousness and health service utilization of the floating population in the Pearl River Delta area: A community perspective. *Journal of Public Management, 11*(4), 125–135.

Zhai, Z., & Duan, C. (2006). *China's migration at the turn of centuries*. Beijing: China Population Publishing House.

Zhang, C. (2011). Empirical analysis on impact of health change on labor supply and income. *Economic Review* (4), 79–88.

Zhang, Q. (1988). Issues on migration and the concept of migrants. *Population Studies* (3), 17–18.

Zhao, H. (2015). The wage disparity between migrants and urban residents: Analysis based on occupational segregation. *World Economic Papers* (2), 91–108.

Zheng, L., Hu, R., Dong, Z., & Hao, Y. (2018). Comparing the needs and utilization of health services between urban residents and rural-to-urban migrants in China from 2012 to 2016. *BMC Health Services Research, 18,* e717.

Zheng, Z., & Lian, P. (2006). Health vulnerability among temporary migrants in urban China. *China Labor Economics, 1*(1), 82–93.

Zhou, H. (2012). Measurement and theoretical perspectives of immigrant assimilation in China. *Population Studies, 36*(3), 27–37.

Chapter 2
Utilization of Basic Public Health Services Among Internal Migrants

Yanqun Liu and Yani Hu

1 Introduction

Undergoing an overwhelming urbanization, there are a huge number of internal migrants in China, which reached 241 million and accounted for about 18% of Chinese total population at the end of 2018 (National Bureau of Statistics, 2019). Migration is a phenomenon of human movement within a geopolitical unit (Gans, 2007; Molloy, Smith, & Wozniak, 2011). In the unique Chinese settings, it refers to a group of people who reside at their residence but are not considered as members of the local official census count (Liu, Wang, Lu, & Liu, 2014). Due to the economic reform that creates abundant employment opportunities, internal migrants have been migrating from poor, remote inlands to rich parts of China since 1979 (Zhu, 2003). Huge waves of internal migrants have not only brought massive labor out of rural areas, but also contributed to the economic growth of host regions. It is estimated that migrant workers have dedicated 16% of Chinese gross domestic product (GDP) growth in the past three decades (Brown & Krasteva, 2013).

However, the large-scale migrant population faces significant challenges. First, internal migrants do not have local household registration (*hukou*). As a permanent household registration system, *hukou* ties citizens' access to services according to their *hukou* location and *hukou* classification (rural vs. urban vs. resident) (Wu & Treiman, 2004). *Hukou* is directly linked with state-funded welfares and social benefits, such as job security, insurances, health care services, housing and child education (Mou, Griffiths, Fong, & Dawes, 2015; Wang, Zuo, & Ruan, 2002). However, the social welfare and healthcare benefits in urban areas are only available to local residents with registered *hukou* (Jin, Hou, & Zhang, 2016). The transfer of *hukou* from rural to urban or from one place to another is difficult for Chinese (Liang, Messener, Chen, & Huang, 2013). Thus, the structure of urban-rural segregation

Y. Liu (✉) · Y. Hu
School of Health Sciences, Wuhan University, Wuhan, China
e-mail: liuyanqun1984@163.com

P. Wang (ed.), *The Health Status of Internal Migrants in China*,
https://doi.org/10.1007/978-981-15-4415-6_2

system limits the public health services utilization of internal migrants (Sun, Chen, & Chan, 2016). Second, most internal migrants are less educated, and few of them can get work-skill training. Consequently, a large number of migrants own dangerous and low-paying jobs in the area of transportation, manufacturing and construction (Wang et al., 2014). The disparities in socioeconomic status (SES) and health awareness between the natives and migrants make the latter face more health risks (Li, Chang, Ji, Shi, & Wang, 2012; Wang et al., 2009).

It is fortunate that these challenges for migrants have drawn significant attention (Zhao et al., 2014). Since 2014, the central government of China has begun to use resident *hukou* to replace agricultural and non-agricultural *hukou*. Also, four basic medical insurances, including New Rural Cooperative Medical Insurance (NRCMI, covering rural areas), Urban-Rural Residence Medical Insurance (URRMI), Urban Residence Medical Insurance (URMI, covering urban areas) and Urban Employee Medical Insurance (UEMI, covering employers), are required to cover 95% of the total population in China. The new policy increases the proportion of internal migrants participating in medical insurance. In 2015, nearly 90% migrants participated in at least one kind of medical insurance, which was 21% higher than in 2011 (Wang, 2016).

China is also on the way to the equalization of public health services (Gong et al., 2012), and the national program of basic public health services is one major project for health equalization. There are 14 health service items in this project, including the establishment of health record (HR), health education (HE), health management for children/the maternal/the elderly, reports and coping strategies of infectious diseases and emergency public health incidents (Government, 2011). Chinese internal migrants usually have a low utilization level of basic public health services and poor health status (Zhang, Liu, & Li, 2013). The failure to provide effective basic public health services for this unique group will hinder the equalization of basic public health services in China (Zhu, Ding, Gu, Guo, & Li, 2013). Thus, it is of great significance to perfect the public health service system and improve the quality of basic public health services for the internal migrants.

Nevertheless, there are numerous problems in the promotion of equalization of basic public health services, such as lack of input from governments, low-quality services, lack of effective coordination linkage mechanisms and low-efficiency service teams (Wang, 2017). From the perspective of financing, the distribution arrangement of public health services based on the number of permanent residents provides an institutional space for local governments to avoid the responsibility of the basic public health services for migrant population. This also leads to the phenomenon of "fall between two stools" in the financing of basic public health services, which hugely restricts the equalization of basic public health service supply among Chinese internal migrants (Duan, Ying, & Zhou, 2016).

HR and HE are two vital tools to provide high-quality health care services for all residences in the community. HR has been promoted to establish since 2009, including paper and electronic HR. Groups that HR focuses on include children (0–6 years old), maternal women, older adults, and people with chronic diseases, serious mental health problems, and tuberculosis. By contrast, HE provides a basis for safe, effective and convenient health services to improve residents' health consciousness, self-care abilities and diseases prevention. It covers many topics, such as nutrition, smoking, reproduction, occupational diseases, chronic diseases, tuberculosis, sexually transmitted diseases (STD)/HIV/AIDS, and mental health problems. Various approaches are used to attract people involving in HE, including lecture, books/magazines/VCD, broadcast/TV programs, chart tools of cellphone, face-to-face counselling, the Internet, and public health activities.

There were articles reporting a high ratio of HR establishment (Bian, Wang, Wang, & Feng, 2014; Huang et al., 2015) or high receiving rate of HE among local residents (Liu, Wang, Gong, Liu, & Chen, 2016). Prior studies mainly focus on the utilization of health and family planning services such as medical insurance, hospital medical treatment and hospital delivery among Chinese internal migrants (Guo & Hu, 2013; Liu, Liu, Wang, & Chen, 2014; Liu et al., 2016; Wang, Guo, Li, Shen, & Liu, 2016; Yin, Xu, & Zheng, 2017), as well as the demand, supply, intervention effect and utilization status of HE (Li et al., 2012; Li, Chai, Sun, & Cheng, 2014; Li, Tian, Chen, & Sun, 2012; Lv et al., 2009; Xu, Fu, & Wan, 2014). However, limited studies have examined the utilization status of HR and HE, as well as their influencing factors, in Chinese internal migrants. It is reported that many individual characteristics are related to the utilization of basic public health services in internal migrants, such as sex, *hukou*, range of migration, work status and household expenditure (Jiang, Zhao, & Shi, 2015). Also, poor health awareness and few access to health resources are important adverse factors of utilization of basic public health services in internal migrants (Guo, Weng, & Zhou, 2014).

Therefore, the purpose of this study was to describe the utilization of HR and HE in Chinese internal migrants and explore the influencing factors of HR and HE.

2 Data and Methods

2.1 Data Source

The data used were from the China Migrant Dynamic Survey (CMDS) of 2015, as well as the data from CMDS in Hubei Province during 2013–2018. CMDS 2015 was conducted in May and June, 2015, with all investigators trained. A multi-stratified, multi-stage and Probability Proportionate to Size (PPS) Sampling design was used, and a total of 206,000 internal migrants (age $\geq$ 15) were investigated in 2015. CMDS 2015 covered four main aspects, including household information, employment, basic public health and family planning services, and medical and health services for the elderly. In this study, there were 10 questionnaires of missing values screened out from 206,000 samples, then 4693 (age $\geq$ 60) questionnaires were excluded; thus, a total of 201,297 samples were used.

CMDS 2013–2018 in Hubei Province was used to analyze the temporal and spatial trends of the utilization of basic public health services in internal migrants, for basic public health service variables were not included in CMDS 2009–2012. From 2013 to 2015, 5999 migrants, 5998 migrants and 6000 migrants in Hubei Province were investigated, respectively, and 5000 migrants were investigated each year from 2016 to 2018. From 2013 to 2014, the survey participants were migrants aged 15–59 who have lived in Hubei Province for no less than one month but had no local *hukou*. From 2015 to 2018, the survey participants were migrants aged 15 or over who have lived in Hubei Province for no less than one month but had no local *hukou*. Since the questionnaire in 2013 only involved the establishment of HR, this paper used the data from 2013 to 2018 to analyze the establishment of HR and its influencing factors, and used the data from 2014 to 2018 to analyze HE receiving and its influencing factors. In multivariate analysis, as employment situation was used, migrants without job were excluded. Therefore, the sample size for HR analysis was 26,670, and the sample size for HE analysis was 21,863.

2.2 Variables

HR and HE were used as dependent variables. For HR, the question was “Have you established residences' health records in the local area?”; for health education, the question was “Have you had access to health knowledge at the local community in the past year?”. Independent variables included sex, age, education, marital status, *hukou*, medical insurance, family monthly income, work status, range of migration, and time of migration.

2.3 Methods

Statistical Package for the Social Sciences (SPSS) version 22.0 was used to analyze the data. Descriptive statistical analysis was conducted to describe the utilization of HR and HE. Chi square test was used to examine group differences in HR and HE. The logistic regression model was used to analyze the influencing factors of HR/HE utilization in Chinese internal migrants. The significance level was set as 0.05.

3 Results

3.1 *Basic Information*

3.1.1 CMDS 2015

A total of 33,081 (16.4%) respondents established HR in local areas, but 168,216 (83.6%) respondents reported no HR in local areas, in which 28.4% of them (57,252) never heard of HR, 26.1% of them (52,603) knew this public health service, and 29.0% of them (58,361) were unclear about HR. For medical insurance, the respondents that participated in NRCMI, URRMI, URMI, UEMI and FMS were 136,209 (67.7%), 8370 (4.2%), 11,549 (5.7%), 35,996 (17.9%) and 264 (0.1%), respectively. Furthermore, for NRCMI, 96.6% (n = 131,620) participants were taken up in their *hukou* registration, 81.0% (n = 6781) for URRMI, 50.5% (n = 5836) for URMI; but for UEMI, 88.9% (n = 32,007) participants were taken up in local areas, and 63.6% (n = 168) for FMS (Table 1). A total of 185,265 (92.0%) respondents received HE in the past one year, most of them received the HE related to reproduction (67.5%), nutrition (65.1%), smoking (61.0%) and STD/HIV/AIDS (56.8%) (see Fig. 1), and propaganda column and broadcast/TV programs were two preferences to receive HE for the respondents (see Fig. 2).

3.1.2 CMDS 2013–2018 in Hubei Province

For the migrants surveyed in Hubei Province during 2013–2018, more than 80.0% of them lived in cities; there were almost equal numbers of male and female migrants; most migrants were 25–34 years old (39.3%–42.5%), and migrants aged over 45 gradually increased from 2013 to 2018. Most migrants received junior high school education, and migrants received college or above education gradually increased from 2013 to 2018. Most respondents were rural-to-urban migrants and had been married. Most migrants migrated within their own provinces. More details can be seen in Table 2.

3.2 *Group Disparities in the Utilization of HR and HE*

Table 3 shows the group disparities in the utilization of HR and HE. Chi square test shows that there were significant differences in the utilization of HR and HE between/among groups with different sex, age, *hukou*, education, migration time, family monthly income and medical insurance ($p < 0.001$). That is to say, males, younger migrants, migrants with agricultural *hukou*, less education, shorter migration

Table 1 Demographic characteristics of Chinese internal migrants: CMDS 2015

Variables	n	%
Sex		
Male	106,454	52.9
Female	94,843	47.1
Age (year)		
15–29	77,109	38.3
30–44	91,310	45.4
45–59	32,878	16.3
Hukou		
Agricultural	169,377	84.1
Non-agricultural	29,085	14.4
Resident	2835	1.4
Education		
Primary school or below	28,898	14.4
Junior high school	102,598	51.0
Senior high school	44,208	22.0
College or above	25,593	12.7
Marital status		
Single or divorce	42650	21.2
Married	158647	78.8
Duration of migration (year)		
Less than 1	22,650	11.3
1–5	102,389	50.9
5–10	47,739	23.7
More than 10	28,519	14.2
Family monthly income (CNY)		
Less than 1000	689	0.3
1000–4999	106,619	53.0
5000–10,000	79,642	39.6
More than 10,000	14,347	7.1
Medical insurance		
With insurance	186,514	92.7
Without insurance	14,783	7.3

duration, moderate family income and migrants without medical insurance were more likely to establish HR. By contrast, females, younger migrants, migrants with resident *hukou*, more education, longer migration duration, more family income and medical insurance were more likely to receive HE.

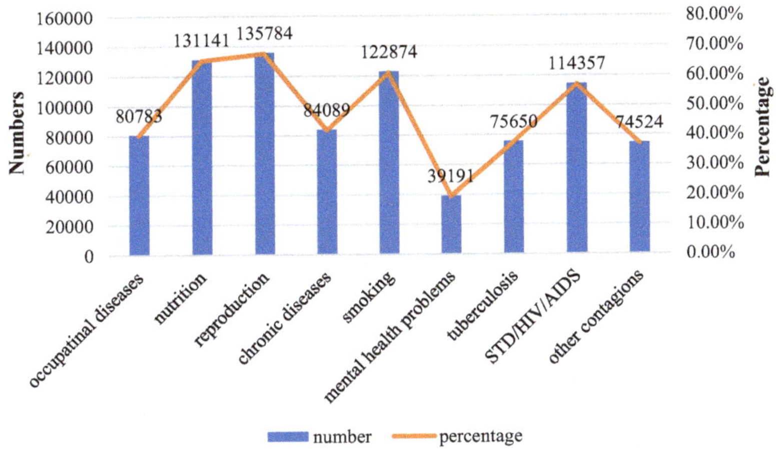

Fig. 1 Numbers and percentage of migrants receiving HE (n = 201,297)

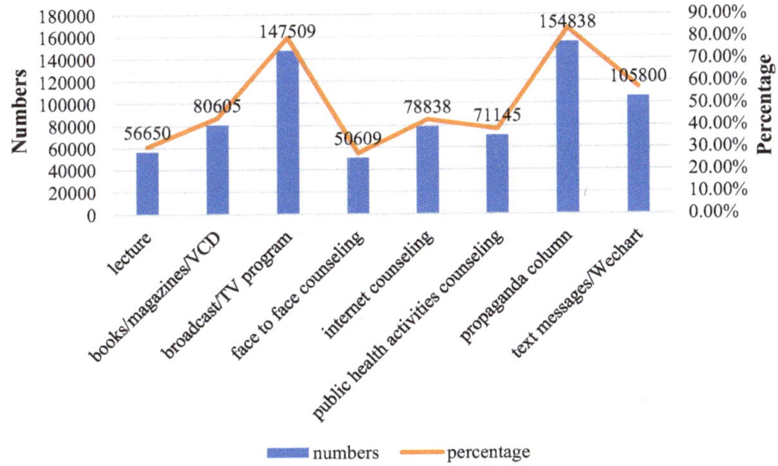

Fig. 2 Numbers and percentages of migrants' preference on HE methods (n = 185,265)

3.3 Temporal Trend of the Utilization of HR and HE in Hubei Province

The establishment rate of HR for the migrants in Hubei Province during 2013–2018 were 27.1%, 45.4%, 73.2%, 82.2%, 46.0%, and 37.1%, respectively ($p < 0.001$, see Table 4). In general, although the establishment rate in 2018 increased by 10.0% compared to 2013, it was a long way to reach the expect target of 80.0% for the standardized electronic establishment rate of HR for migrants in 2020 proposed by the central government of China.

Table 2 Demographic characteristics of Chinese internal migrants in Hubei Province: 2013–2018

Group		2013	2014	2015	2016	2017	2018
		n (%)	n (%)	n (%)	n (%)	n (%)	n (%)
Sex	Male	3092(51.5)	3558(59.3)	3055(50.9)	2586(51.7)	2460(49.2)	2492(49.8)
	Female	2907(48.5)	2440(40.7)	2945(49.1)	2414(48.3)	2540(50.8)	2508(50.2)
Age	15–24	940(15.7)	912(15.2)	879(14.7)	668(13.4)	498(10.0)	475(9.5)
	25–34	2361(39.3)	2485(41.4)	2434(40.6)	2125(42.5)	2071(41.4)	1999(40.0)
	35–44	1993(33.2)	1750(29.2)	1695(28.3)	1354(27.1)	1382(27.6)	1322(26.4)
	45–59	705(11.7)	851(14.2)	930(15.5)	795(15.9)	932(18.6)	1055(21.1)
	≥60	–	–	62(1.0)	58(1.2)	117(2.3)	149(3.0)
Education	Primary school or below	456(7.6)	478(8.0)	561(9.4)	451(9.0)	635(12.7)	632(12.6)
	Junior high school	3841(64.0)	3476(58.0)	3252(54.2)	2449(49.0)	2252(45.0)	2118(42.4)
	Senior high school	1384(23.1)	1424(23.7)	1557(26.0)	1411(28.2)	1374(27.5)	1376(27.5)
	College or above	318(5.3)	620(10.3)	630(10.5)	689(13.8)	739(14.8)	874(17.5)
Hukou	Agricultural	5376(89.6)	5260(87.7)	5191(86.5)	4230(84.6)	4175(83.5)	3941(78.8)
	Non-agricultural	623(10.4)	738(12.3)	809(13.5)	770(15.4)	825(16.5)	1059(21.2)
Marital status	Married	5293(88.2)	5259(87.7)	5341(89.0)	4454(89.1)	4505(90.1)	4489(89.8)
	Single or divorce	706(11.8)	739(12.3)	659(11.0)	546(10.9)	495(9.9)	511(10.2)
Range of migration	Interprovincial	1439(24.0)	1490(24.8)	1512(25.2)	1419(28.4)	1402(28.0)	1395(27.9)
	Cross-city within province	2850(47.5)	2180(36.3)	2168(36.1)	1965(39.4)	1876(37.5)	1872(37.4)
	Cross-county within city	1710(28.5)	2328(38.8)	2320(38.7)	1605(32.2)	1722(34.4)	1733(34.7)

Table 3 Group disparities in the utilization of HR and HE: CMDS 2015

Groups		HR	HE
		n (%)	n (%)
Sex*	Male	18,097(17.0)	97,351 (91.4)
	Female	14,984 (15.8)	87,914 (92.7)
Age*	15–29	13,663 (17.7)	71,240 (92.4)
	30–44	14,237 (15.6)	84,372 (92.4)
	45–59	5181 (15.8)	29,653 (90.2)
*Hukou**	Agricultural	28,231 (16.7)	155,420 (91.8)
	Non-agricultural	4458 (15.3)	27,145 (93.3)
	Resident	392 (13.8)	2700 (95.2)
Education*	Primary school or below	4830 (16.7)	25,549 (88.4)
	Junior high school	17,092 (16.7)	94,309 (91.9)
	Senior high school	7325 (16.6)	41,287 (93.4)
	College or above	3834 (15.0)	24,120 (94.2)
Marital status*	Married	47589(30.0)	146345(92.2)
	Single or divorce	10772(25.3)	38920(91.3)
Migration duration*	Less than 1	4301 (19.0)	20,091 (88.7)
	1–5	17,212 (16.8)	94,923 (92.7)
	5–10	7237 (15.2)	44,329 (92.9)
	More than 10	4331 (15.2)	25,922 (90.9)
Family monthly income*	Less than 1000	109 (15.8)	584 (84.8)
	1000–5000	18,617 (17.5)	97,946 (91.9)
	5000–10,000	12,327 (15.5)	73,522 (92.3)
	More than 10,000	2028 (14.1)	13,213 (92.1)
Medical insurance*	With insurance	30,482 (16.3)	172,239 (92.3)
	Without insurance	2599 (17.6)	13,026 (88.1)

Note $*p < 0.001$

Table 4 Establishment of HR among migrants in Hubei Province: 2013–2018

Establishment of HR	2013	2014	2015	2016	2017	2018
	n (%)	n (%)	n (%)	n (%)	n (%)	n (%)
Yes	1628(27.1)	2721(45.4)	4390(73.2)	4112(82.2)	2174(46.0)	1758(37.1)
Never heard	1284(21.4)	801(13.4)	305(5.1)	245(4.9)	1009(21.3)	1564(33.0)
Not but heard	1144(19.1)	1474(24.6)	785(13.1)	330(6.6)	712(15.1)	797(16.8)
Unclear	1943(32.4)	1002(16.7)	518(8.6)	313(6.3)	831(17.6)	618(13.0)

The receiving rate of HE for migrants in Hubei Province during 2014–2018 were 85.7%, 98.1%, 95.9%, 81.9% and 83.7%, respectively ($p < 0.001$, see Table 5). The receiving rate in 2018 decreased by 2.0% compared to 2014, so it was a long way to reach the expect target of 95.0% for the receiving rate of HE for migrants in 2020 proposed by the central government of China.

During 2014–2018, HE in reproductive health and contraception/maternal health child health/eugenics had the highest receiving rate, while HE in affective disorder and mental health had the lowest receiving rate. More details can be seen in Table 5.

For the receiving method of HE, receiving HE by browsing propaganda columns or propaganda materials accounts for the highest proportion. More details can be seen in Table 6.

Table 5 Temporal trend of HE receiving among migrants in Hubei Province: 2014–2018

Type of HE	2014	2015	2016	2017	2018
	n (%)	n (%)	n (%)	n (%)	n (%)
Occupational disease prevention	1863(31.1)	2740(45.7)	2245(44.9)	1940(41.0)	1791(35.8)
AIDS prevention	3015(50.3)	3777(63.0)	3234(64.7)	2188(46.3)	–
Venereal disease prevention	2541(42.4)				–
reproductive health and contraception	4365(72.8)	4872(81.2)	4193(83.9)	3046(64.5)	2476(49.5)
Maternal and child healthcare/eugenics	–			3098(65.6)	
Tuberculosis prevention	1936(32.3)	2755(45.9)	2312(46.2)	1998(42.3)	–
Affective disorder prevention	863(14.4)	1537(25.6)	1242(24.8)	–	–
Chronic disease prevention	2160(36.0)	3107(51.8)	2739(54.8)	2183(46.2)	1518(30.4)
Nutrition health knowledge	3172(52.9)	4490(74.8)	3431(68.6)	–	–
Infectious disease prevention	1817(30.3)	2787(46.5)	–	–	2127(42.5)
Smoking control	–	4193(69.9)	3232(64.6)	2904(61.4)	–
Haze prevention	–	–	1843(36.9)	–	–
Mental health	–	–	–	2154(45.6)	1007(20.1)
Self-rescue in public emergency	–	–	–	2553(54.0)	1639(32.8)
Others	–	–	–	–	694(13.9)

Table 6 Temporal trend of HE receiving methods among migrants in Hubei Province: 2014–2018

Receiving method of HE	2014	2015	2016	2017	2018
	n (%)	n (%)	n (%)	n (%)	n (%)
Lecture	3428(66.7)	2426(41.2)	3270(68.2)	1898(49.0)	1672(40.0)
Book/magazine/VCD	1904(37.1)	2612(44.4)	–	–	–
Broadcast/TV program	3322(64.7)	4746(80.7)	–	–	–
Face to face counseling	1961(38.2)	2183(37.1)	2480(51.7)	1639(42.3)	679(16.2)
Counseling on the Internet	1603(31.2)	2587(44.0)	526(11.0)	1792(46.3)	–
Short message/WeChat	1364(26.5)	3322(56.5)	1049(21.9)		1503(35.9)
Counseling activity	2237(43.5)	3010(51.2)	–	2160(55.8)	1100(26.3)
Propaganda column	4588(89.3)	5322(90.5)	4514(94.1)	3225(83.3)	2512(60.0)
Electronic screen	–	–	2627(54.8)		–
Propaganda material	–	–	4534(94.5)	3467(89.6)	2937(70.2)
Taught by community doctor	–	–	1664(34.7)	–	–
Others	–	–	–	–	647(15.5)

3.4 *Influencing Factors of HR and HE*

Table 7 shows that males, younger migrants, and migrants with non-resident *hukou*, less education, single or divorce shorter migration duration, less family income and no medical insurance were less likely to establish HR. Table 8 shows that females, older and married migrants, and migrants with resident *hukou*, more education, longer migration duration, more family income and medical insurance were more likely to receive HE.

4 Discussion

Although China attaches importance to the equalization of basic public health services and has made great progress in some areas, it is still a huge challenge to achieve health equalization in internal migrants. In the "Thirteenth Five" years project, the coverage ratio of electronic HR is required to reach 90.0% for Chinese residents (PCR, 2017), but this rate among the internal migrants aged 15–59 in 2015 was 16.4% on a national scale, and it was also less than 90.0% in Hubei Province during 2013–2018. Furthermore, the percentage of migrants that had HR decreased year by year from 2016 t0 2018. Lagging information, heavy workload for healthcare staffs and high mobility of internal migrants might simultaneously result in the low utilization level of HR (Song & Li, 2015). It is observed that most migrants reported they

Table 7 Influencing factors of HR: based on the logistic regression model

Variables	Adjust OR	95%CI		*p*-value
Sex (reference: Female)				
Male	0.082	0.865	0.899	< 0.001
Age (reference: 45–59)				
15–29	0.907	0.878	0.937	< 0.001
30–44	0.981	0.954	1.010	0.191
Hukou (reference: Resident)				
Rural	0.716	0.663	0.774	< 0.001
Urban	0.760	0.700	0.824	< 0.001
Education (reference: College or above)				
Lower than middle school	0.731	0.700	0.763	< 0.001
Middle school	0.874	0.845	0.904	< 0.001
High school	0.989	0.955	1.024	0.053
Marriage (reference: Married)				
Single or divorce	0.796	0.774	0.819	< 0.001
Migrant years (reference: More than 10)				
Less than 1	0.674	0.647	0.703	< 0.001
1–5	0.986	0.957	1.016	0.362
5–10	1.058	1.025	1.093	0.001
Family monthly income (reference: More than 10000)				
Less than 1000	0.896	0.742	1.081	0.251
1000–5000	1.269	1.218	1.321	< 0.001
5000–10,000	1.143	1.097	1.190	< 0.001
Medical insurances (reference: with insurance)				
Without insurance	0.725	0.697	0.755	< 0.001

Note CI: confidence interval

did not have access to or heard of HR, and many migrants were not willing to establish HR. Thus, HR was not convenient or attractive for internal migrants, and many migrants did not recognize the importance of HR. By contrast, over 90.0% respondents have received HE in the past one year, which may attributable to its multiple forms (see Fig. 2). However, some problems cannot be ignored, reproductive health, smoking control and STD/HIV/AIDS prevention should be paid special attention to. Mental health problem was also severe in China. There were about 173 million adults having mental health problems, of which 4.3 million were diagnosed with serious mental health problems (Lancet, 2015). Our results indicated the shortage of mental health practitioners (Gao et al., 2010) and serious discrimination in public (Li, Li, Thornicroft, & Huang, 2014), so we suggested an urgent need in policy, media and research for promoting mental health.

Table 8 Influencing factors of HE: based on the logistic regression model

Variables	Adjust OR	95% CI		*p*-value
Sex (reference: female)				
Male	1.198	1.159	1.239	< 0.001
Age (reference: 45–59)				
15–29	0.868	0.823	0.916	< 0.001
30–44	0.867	0.829	0.907	< 0.001
Hukou (reference: Resident)				
Rural	1.165	1.399	1.983	< 0.001
Urban	1.557	1.300	1.864	< 0.001
Education (reference: College or above)				
Lower than middle school	2.078	1.931	2.235	< 0.001
Middle school	1.418	1.331	1.511	< 0.001
High school	1.132	1.059	1.211	< 0.001
Marriage (reference: Married)				
Single or divorce	1.237	1.182	1.295	< 0.001
Migrant years (reference: More than 10)				
Less than 1	1.331	1.254	1.413	< 0.001
1–5	0.874	0.833	0.917	< 0.001
5–10	0.831	0.787	0.877	< 0.001
Family monthly income (reference: More than 10000)				
Less than 1000	1.484	1.192	1.848	< 0.001
1000–5000	0.865	0.810	0.925	< 0.001
5000–10,000	0.900	0.842	0.962	0.002
Medical insurances (reference: with insurance)				
Without insurance	1.592	1.509	1.679	< 0.001

Note CI: confidence interval

The utilization trend of HR and HE in migrant population in Hubei Province is also not satisfactory. For example, the HE receiving rate of migrant population in Hubei Province declined in 2017. The third edition of the national standard for basic public health services published in 2017 has made it more difficult for primary-level medical and health service institutions to carry out HE. Our study showed that migrants received HE mostly through publicity columns and publicity materials, these ways were more simple and feasible, they contained more information and had intuitive contents and visual impacts compared with other ways. With the development of the Internal, more and more migrants prefer to receive HE by Wechat or short message, which has increased from 26.5 % in 2013 to 35.9% in 2018. We also found that reproductive health and contraception, maternal and child health care/eugenics and eugenics received more attention than other HE contents during 2014–2018 in Hubei

Province, one explanation is that the government has emphasized more on reproductive health services and maternal and child health care in recent years (Fan, 2019; Guo et al., 2014; Jiang et al., 2015). However, the level of mental disorders prevention and treatment and mental health education were still low in recent years, which was similar to the status in 2015. The current mental health service capacity and level in China are far from meeting the health needs of residents (Chen & Mei, 2016; Liu, 2013), this may limit the access to mental health education in Chinese internal migrants.

We also found disparities in the utilization of HR and HE on the basis of sex, age, *hukou*, education, migration duration, family income and medical insurance, which were mostly in line with the results from prior studies (Guo, Shao, Fan, Xue, & Wu, 2016; Guo & Huang, 2016; Nie, Shen, & Bao, 2016). Female migrants (Nie et al., 2016), and migrants with more education, more family income (Guo et al., 2016; Nie et al., 2016) and medical insurance (Guo et al., 2016) were more likely to establish HR and receive HE in communities. Previous studies find that older adults prefer to establish HR and receive HE (Guo et al., 2016; Nie et al., 2016), but younger adults were more likely to receive HE and less likely to establish HR in our study. Various accesses to HE receiving (e.g., online access and mobile phone access) are convenient and feasible for younger group, but complex routines, payment of HR and good health may result in the lower likelihood of the young to establish HR. Prior studies suggest that online access (Roblin, Houston, Allison, Joski, & Becker, 2009) and health status (Ancker et al., 2011) significantly influence patients to establish HR.

Some disparities may be caused by the difference in sampling and coding methods. For example, a prior study reports that migration duration only influences the establishment of HR among migrants in Shanghai, China (Nie et al., 2016). The change of relevant policies may also influence the establishment of HR among Chinese internal migrants. Based on the data in CMDS 2014, Nie et al. (2016) found migrants with non-rural *hukou* were more likely to establish HR and receive HE. However, our results showed migrants with resident *hukou* were more likely to establish HR and receive HE. The Urban-rural *hukou* system has limited rural-to-urban migrants to receive basic public health services. Resident *hukou*, which has been conducted since July, 2014, can make migrants share similar welfares as the natives. The policy change has got effects as our research presented, but it is still a long way to run because most migrants are rural-to-urban migrants with rural or agricultural *hukou* in modern China.

In view of the above results, our study tries to put forward some beneficial policy implications to improve the utilization of basic public health services in China. First, the government should attach great importance to the establishment of HR. A coordination mechanism among administrative departments of health and family planning at all levels should be comprehensively established to promote policies conducive to the equal access to basic public health services in migrants and well integrate migrant population into the scope of community health and family planning services. The focus of HR construction should be at the grassroots level. We should take the lead in developing community medical social workers in developed areas and assist community health service centers in carrying out basic public health services

(Yin & Xu, 2018). Second, we should give full play to the effectiveness of HE and promote the combination of medical treatment and prevention. At the same time, the establishment of HR can be combined with female screening for cancer and physical examination to guide them to involve in self-health management. Third, according to the different needs of migrants, multiple and targeted HE contents should be provided for different migrant groups (Xue, Fan, & Guo, 2017). We should pay particular attention to mental health education and strengthen the training of mental health professionals. HE should be conducted in the place with high-density migrants, especially construction sites, factories and communities (Du, Liu, & Cheng, 2011). Finally, traditional HE mode and new media HE mode should be combined to enrich the form of HE. On the basis of traditional methods, new media such as the Internet, WeChat and microblog should be adopted to generate new HE modes; migrants should be fully mobilized, especially the young, to participate in HE so that they can acquire HE information more effectively (Wang, 2011). Simultaneously, mass organizations such as trade unions, communist youth league, women's federations, family planning associations and other non-governmental organizations can be used to increase publicity efforts to make migrant population familiar with the content and process of relevant projects.

This study used a nationally representative sample to explore disparities in the utilization of HR and HE in Chinese internal migrants. It extended previous studies by reporting sex, age, education, *hukou*, marital status, migrant duration, family income and medical insurance disparities, as well as the temporal trend, in the utilization of HR and HE. However, there were limitations in this study. First, migrants with medical insurance were more likely to establish HR and receive HE than those without medical insurance, but we did not compare differences among groups with various medical insurances. Second, other potential disparities, such as personal income and regional, were not examined in this study. Finally, the data from Hubei Province rather than nationally representative data were used to describe the temporal trend in the utilization of HR and HE. Further studies should discuss these issues.

5 Conclusion

The access to HR and HE of mental health problems was poor, topic of mental health problems was the least attendance in HE; female migrants, married migrants and migrants with more education, resident *hukou*, more family monthly income and medical insurance were more likely to establish HR and receive HE; older adults were more likely to establish HR while the younger group was more likely to receive HE. More convenient and feasible routines of HR should be taken into consideration to attract migrants on the basis of different characteristics. Policymakers and communities should strengthen advocacy on mental health and improve migrants' initiative and willingness to participate in these health activities.

References

Ancker, J. S., Barrón, Y., Rockoff, M. L., Hauser, D., Pichardo, M., Szerencsy, A., et al. (2011). Use of an electronic patient portal among disadvantaged populations. *Journal of General Internal Medicine, 26*(10), 1117–1123.

Bian, L., Wang, Y., Wang, M., & Feng, Y. (2014). Health records defects of community health files and countermeasures. *Chinese General Practice, 17*(16), 1834–1836.

Brown, E., & Krasteva, A. (2013). *Migrants and refugees: Equitable education for displaced populations*. Charlotte: IAP.

Chen, Z., & Mei, Z. (2016). Influence of migrant population on social economic development and status quo of basic public health services in China. *Chinese Remedies & Clinics, 16*(5), 609–612.

Du, X., Liu, E., & Cheng, S. (2011). Characteristic analysis of newly smear-positive tuberculosis patients among registered floating population in 2010. *Chinese Journal of Tuberculosis Prevention, 99*(8), 461–465.

Duan, D., Ying, Y., & Zhou, J. (2016). A study on the financing mechanism of prompting the equalized supply of basic public health services for China' migrant population. *Population & Economics* (4), 34–44.

Fan, X. (2019). Health status of Chinese migrants: Problems and countermeasures. *Macroeconomic Management* (4), 42–47.

Gans, P. (2007). *Internal migration patterns in the EU and the future population development of large cities in Germany*. Chile: Santiago de.

Gao, X., Jackson, T., Chen, H., Liu, Y., Wang, R., Qian, M., et al. (2010). There is a long way to go: A nationwide survey of professional training for mental health practitioners in China. *Health Policy, 95*(1), 74–81.

Gong, P., Liang, S., Carlton, E. J., Jiang, Q., Wu, J., Wang, L., et al. (2012). Urbanisation and health in China. *Lancet, 379*(9818), 843–852.

Government, C. N. H. a. F. P. C. C. (2011). National Basic Public Health Services Specification. Retrieved from http://www.nhfpc.gov.cn/zwgk/wtwj/201304/cb5978bb42814451a26e5c97dd855254.shtml.

Guo, J., Shao, F., Fan, H., Xue, L., & Wu, Y. (2016). Analysis on the access to the basic public health care services and influencing factors among migrants. *Chinese Journal of Health Policy, 9*(8), 75–82.

Guo, J., Weng, H., & Zhou, Q. (2014). Status quo and determinants on basic public health services of floating population. *Chinese Journal of Health Policy, 7*(8), 51–56.

Guo, L., & Hu, H. (2013). Study on the impact of the new rural cooperative medical system on the utilization of health services for farmers. *Soft Science of Health, 27*(12), 723–729.

Guo, X., & Huang, L. (2016). The situation and influence factors of health records of floating population: Based on the National Dynamic Monitoring Data of Floating Population Survey of Sichuan Province in 2014. *Population and Development, 22*(3), 84–89.

Huang, L., Yan, X., Liu, J., Wen, F., Ma, L., & Su, W. (2015). Surveying the status of establishment and management of residents' health records in Sichuan Province. *Chinese Health Service Management, 31*(2), 152–154.

Jiang, T., Zhao, Y., & Shi, Z. (2015). The research on migrant's equalization of public health services quality: Based on the Migrant's Dynamic Monitoring Survey data in 2013. *Journal of Macro-Quality Research, 3*(1), 111–119.

Jin, Y., Hou, Z., & Zhang, D. (2016). Determinants of health insurance coverage among people aged 45 and over in China: Who buys public, private and multiple insurance. *PLoS ONE, 11*(8), e161774.

Lancet. (2015). Mental health in China: What will be achieved by 2020? *Lancet, 385*(9987), 2548.

Li, C., Chang, C., Ji, Y., Shi, Y., & Wang, D. (2012a). Survey on the utilization and satisfaction of public health services among young floating population. *Chinese Journal of Health Education, 28*(6), 434–437.

Li, G., Gao, Y., Qi, Y., Qiu, X., Teng, X., & Pang, Z. (2012b). Evaluation of the effect of health education on health knowledge and behavior of young floating population and on the utilization of health services. *Chinese Journal of Health Education, 28*(2), 138–140.

Li, J., Li, J., Thornicroft, G., & Huang, Y. (2014a). Levels of stigma among community mental health staff in Guangzhou, China. *BMC Psychiatry, 14,* e231.

Li, M., Chai, Y., Sun, J., & Cheng, Y. (2014b). Survey on health status and related knowledge and behavior of floating population. *Chinese Journal of Health Education, 30*(12), 1068–1071.

Li, Z., Tian, B., Chen, J., & Sun, X. (2012c). Survey on knowledge, behavior and needs of tuberculosis prevention and control among floating population in 3 provinces and cities of China. *Chinese Journal of Health Education, 28*(8), 607–610.

Liang, Z., Messener, S. F., Chen, C., & Huang, Y. (2013). The emergence of a new urban China. *Contemporary Sociology, 42,* 860–861.

Liu, D., Liu, H., Wang, H., & Chen, J. (2014a). The present situation and influencing factors of in-hospital delivery of pregnant and lying-in women in floating population. *Chinese Journal of Public Health, 30*(12), 1523–1526.

Liu, D., Wang, H., Gong, S., Liu, H., & Chen, J. (2016). The current situation and influencing factors of repeated participation of floating population in basic medical insurance in China. *Chinese Journal of Public Health, 32*(1), 62–65.

Liu, H., Wang, Q., Lu, Z., & Liu, J. (2014b). Reproductive health service use and social determinants among the floating population: A quantitative comparative study in Guangzhou City. *BMC Health Services Research, 14*(1), e502.

Liu, Y. (2013). The general situation of development, problems and countermeasures about community mental health service in China. *Chinese Journal of Social Medicine, 30*(6), 379–380.

Lv, W., Lin, B., Zhang, K., Liu, T., Liu, Y., Lu, J., et al. (2009). Survey on the cognitive and health education needs of migrant population injuries. *Chinese Journal of Health Education, 25*(12), 900–902.

Molloy, R., Smith, C., & Wozniak, A. (2011). Internal migration in the United States: National Bureau of Economic Research.

Mou, J., Griffiths, S., Fong, H. F., & Dawes, M. (2015). Defining migration and its health impact in China. *Public Health, 129,* (1326–1334).

National Bureau of Statistics. (2019). *China statistical yearbook 2019.* Beijing: China Stastics Press.

Nie, H., Shen, W., & Bao, Y. (2016). Analysis on the establishment of health records and health education status of floating population in Shanghai. *Chinese Journal of General Practice, 14*(1), 101–104.

PCR, T. S. C. o. (2017). The "Thirteen Five" Project for promoting basic public services equalization. Retrieved from http://www.gov.cn/zhengce/content/2017-03/01/content_5172013.htm.

Roblin, D. W., Houston, T. K., Allison, J. J., Joski, P. J., & Becker, E. R. (2009). Disparities in use of a personal health record in a managed care organization. *Journal of the American Medical Informatics Association, 16*(5), 683–689.

Song, Y., & Li, L. (2015). Investigation and analysis of the status and problems of the healthcare archives in floating population. *Archives Science Bulletin* (3), 84–88.

Sun, X., Chen, M., & Chan, K. L. (2016). A meta-analysis of the impacts of internal migration on child health outcomes in China. *BMC Public Health, 16,* e66.

Wang, F., Zuo, X., & Ruan, D. (2002). Rural migrants in Shanghai: Living under the shadow of socialism. *International Migration Review, 36*(2), 520–545.

Wang, H., Guo, W., Li, P., Shen, Q., & Liu, H. (2016). Basic public services of health and family planning for floating population in Shanghai and Guangdong. *Maternal and Child Health Care of China, 31*(10), 2026–2027.

Wang, J.-W., Cui, Z.-T., Ding, N., Zhang, C.-G., Usagawa, T., Berry, H. L., et al. (2014). A qualitative study of smoking behavior among the floating population in Shanghai, China. *BMC Public Health, 14,* e1138.

Wang, J., Gu, S., Zhao, A., Ding, Y., Chen, D., & Wen, D. (2009). Survey on health education needs of migrant workers in Shanghai. *Health Education and Health Promotion, 4*(S1), 11–14.

Wang, P. (2016). *Report on China's migrant population development*. Beijing: China Population Publishing House.
Wang, X. (2011). The role of mobile message in health education communication. *Chinese Journal of Health Education, 27*(4), 311–313.
Wang, X. (2017). Study on the equalization of basic public health services for floating population. *Journal of Tianjin Administration Institute, 19*(3), 3–7.
Wu, X., & Treiman, D. J. (2004). The household registration system and social stratification in China: 1955-1996. *Demography, 41*(2), 363–384.
Xu, Y., Fu, Y., & Wan, Y. (2014). Study on health education for tuberculosis among floating population in Tianjin Binhai New Area. *Chinese Journal of Health Education, 30*(4), 344–346.
Xue, L., Fan, H., & Guo, J. (2017). Study on health education status and influencing factors of floating population. *Chinese Journal of Health Education, 33*(9), 771–774.
Yin, Q., & Xu, Q. (2018). Analysis of the status quo and influencing factors of the establishment of health records for floating population. *Chinese Journal of Public Health, 34*(10), 1351–1355.
Yin, Q., Xu, Q., & Zheng, Y. (2017). Analysis of the current situation and influencing factors of in-patient medical service utilization of floating population. *Chinese Journal of Public Health, 33*(3), 448–451.
Zhang, D., Liu, Y., & Li, W. (2013). Advances in comprehensive strategies of self-health management for the elderly. *Journal of Nursing, 20*(11), 25–27.
Zhao, Y., Kang, B., Liu, Y., Li, Y., Shi, G., Shen, T., et al. (2014). Health insurance coverage and its impact on medical cost: Observations from the floating population in China. *PLoS ONE, 9*(11), e111555.
Zhu, Y. (2003). The floating population's household strategies and the role of migration in China's regional development and integration. *International Journal of Population Geography, 9*(6), 485–502.
Zhu, Y., Ding, Y., Gu, C., Guo, H., & Li, X. (2013). Analysis of community health service needs and utilization of residents in Zhonglou District, Changzhou City, Jiangsu Province in 2010. *Chinese Journal of Health Education, 29*(3), 235–239.

Chapter 3
Association Between Medical Insurance, Migration Direction and Health Seeking Behaviors of Internal Migrants

Jing Liang and Shuqin Wu

1 Introduction

Since the Reform and Opening Up in 1978, some major changes have taken place in China's society and economy, and migrant population have become an important group in China. Internal migrants who do not live in their hometown reached 241 million in 2018, and they usually migrate to richer regions to work for money. This also indirectly realizes the transfer of population among different regions. However, because of the limitation of the household registration system, they have failed to truly melt into the city and realized the "synchronizing citizenization" (Yu & Zhu, 2018). The states of long-term mobility, poor living environment, low occupational status and strong occupational pressure have led to numerous health problems among internal migrants, and they also have less access to local health services (Christian et al., 2015; Colón-Burgos et al., 2014; Huang, Chen, & Pong, 2015; Lam & Johnston, 2012; Liu, Hu, & Mak, 2013; Mou et al., 2009).

Prior studies have shown that the health care utilization level among migrants is lower than that among the natives. For example, the rate of outpatient among migrants to the UK is 38.5%, while it is 43.5% among the UK natives (Saunders et al., 2020); In China, the rate of two-week visits for internal migrants is 8.74%, the rate of two-week untreated cases for them is 38.98% (Li, Gu, Huang, Lv, & Zhang, 2010), only 30% internal migrants choose to go to see a doctor when they are sick, and the rest choose medical treatment or do not take any measures (Liu & Wu, 2012). Although 30% internal migrants go to see a doctor after they are sick, nearly 20% of them prefer to go to primary health institutions and private clinics, and they do not go to high-level medical institutions unless their diseases are serious (Guo, Wang, Yang, Guo, & Li, 2008). Lack of medical insurance, high cost of healthcare and exacting

J. Liang (✉) · S. Wu
School of Health Sciences, Wuhan University, Wuhan, China
e-mail: liang0827@whu.edu.cn

P. Wang (ed.), *The Health Status of Internal Migrants in China*,
https://doi.org/10.1007/978-981-15-4415-6_3

work schedules have limited their access to regular medical services (Hong et al., 2006).

In order to improve the equity of access to health services, China's medical security system has undergone some major changes. The Urban Employee Basic Medical Insurance (UEBMI) was established in China in 1998 (Liu, 2002), the New Rural Cooperative Medical Scheme (NCMS) was introduced in rural areas in 2003, and the Urban Resident Basic Medical Insurance (URBMI) was implemented in urban areas in 2008. The coverage of these three major basic health insurances in China increased rapidly from 29.7% in 2003 to 95% in 2011 (Meng et al., 2012). However, there are significant differences in insurance coverage, treatment level and reimbursement ratio among different types of medical insurance. UEBMI is significantly superior to URBMI and NCMS in these respects. For example, the average reimbursement ratio of UEBMI is about 70%, but it is only about 50% for URBMI and NCMS (Sun, Deng, Xiong, & Tang, 2014; Ye et al., 2013).

Many prior studies have discussed the positive effect of medical insurance system on the utilization of health services, especially UEBMI (Han & Meng, 2019). UEBMI can help residents reduce the burden of expenses and improve the probability to acquaint high-quality health services. Although most internal migrants in China have NCMS, they have a lower take-up proportion in UEBMI. As China's medical insurance is managed on a regional basis (Jiang, 2016), internal migrants will face some problems caused by seeking medical treatment in non-resident places, such as the complicated procedures of reimbursement and low reimbursement ratio. These problems may exacerbate the health inequalities existed, which make internal migrants unwilling to be treated if they have minor diseases and afraid of treatment if they have serious diseases.

Numerous studies have studied social and personal influencing factors of health seeking behaviors among internal migrants (Tang, Li, He, & Zhang, 2016). Social environment, social support, medical security, and medical service system are considered main social factors that have influences on migrants' health seeking behaviors. The medical technology, price level and geographical accessibility of medical service institutions are important factors affecting residents' health seeking behaviors. Age, gender, education, occupation, income, individual health status, health cognition and other basic attributes are also considered and widely investigated as factors affecting people's health seeking behaviors. For internal migrants, their unique migration characteristics, including the range, duration and other features of migration, make the influence of multiple factors on their health seeking behaviors more complicated (Liu, 2011). Guo and her colleagues found that migration duration is a main factor affecting the utilization of health services among internal migrants (Guo, Zhou, Guo, & Wu, 2015).

In addition to the range and duration of migration, the direction of migration should also attract more attention. Eastern China has a higher level of socioeconomic development than Middle and Western China, so most internal migrants migrate from Middle and Western China to Eastern China (Zhai, Wang, & Shi, 2019). However, different migrant directions may lead to different income and access to health care resources. Some studies found Eastern China has more health resources and return on income than Middle and Western China (Ma, Chen, & Shi, 2018; Zhang, Xu, Ren, Sun, & Liu, 2017), which have an impact on migrants' health seeking behaviors.

Health seeking behavior reflects people' need and utilization of medical and health care resources, which is closely related to their health and quality of life (Shen, Shi, Wang, & Sun, 2019). Taking migration direction and medical insurance into account, we focused on investigating the current situation of health seeking behaviors among internal migrants and its influencing factors, which can help reform and perfect the medical health security system and improve their health seeking behaviors.

2 Data and Methods

2.1 Data Sources

The China Migrants Dynamic Survey (CMDS) was conducted by the National Health and Family Planning Commission of China. The first survey was conducted in 2009, followed by one per year until 2018. CMDS was an open access and nationally representative cross-sectional survey, which aimed to investigate internal migrants aged 15 and above who did not have local household registration (*hukou*) and had been living in local residence for no less than one month. The sample was drawn using a stratified multi-stage random sampling method with the Probability Proportional to Size (PPS) approach. The survey covered 348 cities from 31 provincial units in mainland China. Neighborhoods in urban or suburban areas were randomly selected using the PPS approach within each city, and a total of 10,300 communities nationwide were investigated. In each selected neighborhood, a total of 20 migrants were randomly selected, and the survey was conducted through face-to-face interviews. All participants provided their informed consent for inclusion before they participated in the survey.

The data used in this study were from CMDS in 2014. In this study, we focused on the migrants who had been hospitalized within 12 months and had medical insurance, with a sample size of 5590 in total. There were 90.52% of internal migrants who migrated from western regions to other regions. Therefore, in order to keep the homogeneity of the sample, migrants who had *hukou* of western regions were selected as our study subjects (n = 5060). The survey covered basic demographic information of internal migrants, range and direction of migration, employment and social security, income, housing expenditure, essential public health services, management of marriage and family planning services, children mobility and education, and psychological culture.

2.2 Main Outcome

The health seeking behaviors of internal migrants are measured using hospitalization level and the reimbursement ratio. The question "Which level of hospital were you in when you were sick in the last year?" included the choice of "township health centers", "community health service centers", "county and district public hospitals", "private hospitals", "prefecture-level public hospitals" and "provincial (autonomous regions, municipalities) or above public hospitals". In this study, we divided it into three categories: "public hospitals at county/district level or below" (including "township hospitals", "community health service centers" and "county and district public hospitals"), "public hospitals at prefecture-level or above" (including "prefecture-level public hospitals" and "provincial (autonomous region, municipality) or above public hospitals") and "private hospitals". The reimbursement ratio is based on the question "How much did your last hospitalization medical cost" and "How much did your basic medical insurance reimburse".

2.3 Explanatory Variables

Medical insurance and migration direction among internal migrants were used as explanatory variables in this study. Medical insurance was divided into three categories: UEBMI, NCMS and URBMI. China were divided into three regions based on the geographical location and level of economic development, namely eastern region, central region and western region. Therefore, migration direction was divided into three categories: West–East, West–Central and West–West.

2.4 Control Variables

Control variables included demographic characteristic, socioeconomic status and others. Demographic characteristics included gender, marriage status (married vs. unmarried), and age (a continuous variable). Socioeconomic status were measured by education (primary school and below, junior high school, senior high school, college degree and above), *hukou* (agricultural vs. non-agricultural), race (han nationality vs. minority) and residence (village committee vs. resident committee).

2.5 Data Analysis

Descriptive analysis was used to describe the basic information of variables used. We used multinomial logistic models to analyze influence factors of the hospitalization level in all sample and three subgroups divided by migration direction. The formula is as follows:

$$Ln\left[\frac{\pi_j}{\pi_J}\right] = \alpha + \beta_1 x_1 + \beta_2 x_2 + \beta_3 x_i$$

Among them, $Ln\left[\frac{\pi_j}{\pi_J}\right]$ is the log relative risk for internal migrants to choose hospitalization level j and hospitalization level J (base outcome); α is a constant term; β_1, β_2, β_3 are partial regression coefficients; x_1 is migration direction; x_2 is medical insurance; x_i is the control variable (include gender, marriage status, age, education, *hukou* status, race and residence).

We also used multivariate linear regression to analyze influence factors of reimbursement ratio in all samples and above three subgroups. All statistical analyses were conducted using Stata version 12.0. $\alpha = 0.05$ was set as the statistically significant level.

3 Results

As shown in Table 1, a total of 5060 internal migrants were analyzed, of which 75.45% were female, with an average age of 32.07 years old. Most of them had a

Table 1 Characteristics of internal migration in 2014 (n = 5060)

Variables	M/n	SD (%)	Variables	M/n	SD (%)
Hospitalization level			*Education*		
County/district level or below public hospitals	2717	53.60	Primary school or below	685	13.54
Prefecture-level or above public hospitals	2047	40.45	Junior high school	2406	47.55
Private hospitals	301	5.95	Senior high school	1028	20.32
Reimbursement ratio	0.27	0.33	College or above	941	18.60
Migration direction			*Race*		
West–East	2200	43.48	Han nationality	4600	90.91
West–Central	1114	22.02	Minority	460	9.09
West–West	1746	34.51	*Marital status*		
Medical insurance			Married	4793	94.72
NCMS	3477	68.72	Unmarried	267	5.28
UEBMI	1156	22.85	*Residence*		
URBMI	427	8.44	Resident committee	3576	70.67
Gender			Village committee	1484	29.33
Male	1242	24.55	*Hukou*		
Female	3818	75.45	Agricultural	4231	83.62
Age	32.07	8.52	Non-agricultural	829	16.38

Note % meant percentage. M: mean, n: number, SD: standard deviation

Table 2 Influence of migration direction and medical insurance on hospitalization level

County/district level or below public hospitals (base outcome)		Prefecture-level or above public hospitals	Private hospitals
		RRR(95%CI)	RRR(95%CI)
Migration direction	West–East	1.000	1.000
	West–Central	2.030(1.725–2.388)*	1.641(1.194–2.257)*
	West–West	1.826(1.582–2.107)*	1.401(1.048–1.872)*
Medical insurance	NCMS	1.000	1.000
	UEBMI	1.263(1.063–1.499)*	1.009(0.703–1.448)
	URBMI	0.916(0.730–1.151)	0.604(0.356–1.025)
Residence	Resident committee	1.000	1.000
	Village committee	0.663(0.576–0.762)*	0.605(0.454–0.808)*
Gender	Male	1.000	1.000
	Female	1.162(0.995–1.357)	0.740(0.549–0.997)*
Age		1.031(1.022–1.039)*	0. 399(0.976–1.010)
Race	Han nationality	1.000	1.000
	Minority	0.959(0.775–1.187)	0.745(0.468–1.187)
Education	Primary school or below	1.000	1.000
	Junior high school	1.230(1.009–1.499)*	1.061(0.722–1.561)
	Senior high school	1.596(1.269–2.007)*	0.797(0.498–1.277)
	College or above	1.896(1.462–2.460)*	0.842(0.490–1.448)
Hukou	Agricultural	1.000	1.000
	Non-agricultural	1.436(1.186–1.738)*	1.457(0.971–2.185)
Marriage status	Married	1.000	1.000
	Unmarried	1.132(0.856–1.496)	1.136(0.671–1.922)
Constant term		0.130(0.084–0.200)*	0.168 (0.072–0.390)*

Note $*p < 0.05$, RRR: relative-risk ratio, CI: confidence interval

junior high school education (47.55%) and a senior high school education (20.32%). Migrants with agricultural *hukou* accounted for 83.62%, 90.91% of them belonged to Han nationality, 94.72% of them were married, and 70.67% of them lived in resident committees. Internal migrants from the west to the east accounted for 43.48%, and it was 22.02% for those from the west to the central and 34.51% for those from the west to the west. A total of 68.72% internal migrants participated in NCMS, and it was 22.85% for the UEBMI and 8.44% for the URBMI.

A total of 53.60% internal migrants chose to be hospitalized in public hospitals at county/district level or below, 40.45% internal migrants chose to be hospitalized in public hospitals at prefecture-level or above, while only 5.95% internal migrants chose to go to private hospitals. The average reimbursement ratio for hospitalization was 27.00%.

The influencing factors of hospitalization level were shown in Table 2. After demographic characteristic and socioeconomic status were controlled for, compared with hospitalization in county/district level or below public hospitals, internal migrants migrating from the west to the central (RRR = 2.030, 95%CI: 1.725–2.388), migrating from the west to the west (RRR = 1.826, 95%CI: 1.582–2.107), having UEBMI (RRR = 1.263, 95%CI: 1.063–1.499), being older (RRR = 1.031, 95%CI: 1.022–1.039), having more education (junior high school: RRR = 1.230, 95%CI: 1.009–1.499; senior high school: RRR = 1.596, 95%CI: 1.269–2.007; college or above: RRR = 1.896, 95%CI: 1.462–2.460) and having non-agricultural *hukou* (RRR = 1.436, 95%CI: 1.186–1.738) were more likely to go to hospitalized in prefecture-level or above public hospitals, while internal migrants living in village committee (RRR = 0.663, 95%CI: 0.576–0.762) were less likely to go to hospitalized in the prefecture-level or above public hospitals.

After demographic characteristic and socioeconomic status were controlled for, compared with hospitalized in county/district level or below public hospitals, internal migrants migrating from the west to the central (RRR = 1.641, 95%CI: 1.194–2.257), migrating from the west to the west (RRR = 1.401, 95%CI: 1.048–1.872) were more likely to go to hospitalized in the private hospitals, while internal migrants living in village committee (RRR = 0.605, 95%CI:0.454–0.808) and being female (RRR = 0.740, 95%CI: 0.549–0.997) were less likely to go to hospitalized in the private hospitals.

Table 3 showed the effect of medical insurance on the choice of hospitalization level among migrants with different migration directions. The results showed that, with other influencing factors controlled for, different types of medical insurance had no significant association with the choice of hospitalization level. However, in the subgroup of West-West direction, compared with internal migrants participated in NCMS, the ratio of county/district or below public hospitals and private hospitals was higher in those with UEBMI (RRR = 1.633, 95%CI: 1.174–2.273).

Table 4 showed the influencing factors of reimbursement ratio among internal migrants. In all samples, with demographic characteristic and socioeconomic status controlled for, the average medical insurance reimbursement ratio in internal migrants from the west to the west was 0.041 unit higher ($p < 0.05$) than that in migrants from the west to the east. The average reimbursement ratio in internal migrants with URBMI was 0.043 unit higher than that in internal migrants with NCMS ($p < 0.05$), while the average reimbursement ratio in internal migrants with UEBMI was 0.268 unit higher than that in internal migrants with NCMS ($p < 0.05$). Increasing age by 1 year increases the ratio by 0.3%. Compared with primary school and below, the higher the education level, the higher the ratio (senior high school: $\beta = 0.035$, $p < 0.05$; college or above: $\beta = 0.047$, $p < 0.05$).

We performed a similar multivariate linear regression analysis separately in above three subgroups: the west to the east, the west to the central, and the west to the west (see Table 4). Among internal migrants from the west to the east, the average medical insurance reimbursement ratio in internal migrants with UEBMI was 0.274 unit ($p < 0.05$) higher than that in migrants with NCMS. Among internal migrants from the west to the central, the average medical insurance reimbursement ratio in internal migrants with UEBMI was 0.252 unit ($p < 0.05$) higher than that in migrants with

Table 3 Influence of medical insurance on hospitalization level in different migrant directions

County/district level or below public hospitals (base outcome)		Prefecture-level or above public hospitals			Private hospitals		
		West-East	West-Central	West-West	West-East	West-Central	West-West
		RRR(95%CI)	RRR(95%CI)	RRR(95%CI)	RRR(95%CI)	RRR(95%CI)	RRR(95%CI)
Medical insurance	NCMS	1.000	1.000	1.000	1.000	1.000	1.000
	UEBMI	1.170(0.927–1.475)	1.011(0.655–1.562)	1.633(1.174–2.273)*	0.991(0.608–2.616)	0.605(0.225–1.619)	1.521(0.780–2.969)
	URBMI	1.034(0.680–1.572)	1.038(0.666–1.619)	0.882(0.619–1.257)	0.577(0.201–1.661)	0.648(0.234–1.792)	0.642(0.289–1.427)
Residence	Resident committee	1.000	1.000	1.000	1.000	1.000	1.000
	Village committee	0.506(0.408–0.627)	0.706(0.508–0.981)*	0.861(0.686–1.082)	0.872(0.582–1.305)	0.497(0.238–1.037)	0.334(0.182–0.613)*
Gender	Male	1.000	1.000	1.000	1.000	1.000	1.000
	Female	1.227(0.938–1.604)	1.136(0.830–1.553)	1.126(0.884–1.436)	0.593 (0.367–0.959)*	1.054(0.559–1.986)	0.760(0.466–1.237)
Age		1.037(1.022–1.052)*	1.031(1.014–1.048)*	1.025(1.011–1.039)*	0.999(0.971–1.027)	0.990(0.956–1.025)	0.989(0.961–1.018)
Race	Han nationality	1.000	1.000	1.000	1.000	1.000	1.000
	Minority	1.071(0.700–1.638)	0.762(0.390–1.490)	0.912(0.699–1.189)	1.371(0.681–2.758)	0.000(0.000–0.000)	0.651(0.345–1.231)
Education	Primary school or below	1.000	1.000	1.000	1.000	1.000	1.000
	Junior high school	1.120(0.787–1.594)	1.430(0.921–2.218)	1.222(0.916–1.629)	0.831(0.456–1.517)	0.850(0.379–1.906)	1.545(0.811–2.944)
	Senior high school	1.578(1.060–2.349)*	1.798(1.102–2.933)*	1.502(1.053–2.142)*	0.543(0.249–1.181)	0.644(0.248–1.675)	1.282(0.588–2.795)

(continued)

Table 3 (continued)

County/district level or below public hospitals (base outcome)		Prefecture-level or above public hospitals			Private hospitals		
		West-East	West-Central	West-West	West-East	West-Central	West-West
		RRR(95%CI)	RRR(95%CI)	RRR(95%CI)	RRR(95%CI)	RRR(95%CI)	RRR(95%CI)
	College or above	1.757(1.147–2.692)*	2.388(1.302–4.381)*	1.715(1.136–2.590)*	0.787(0.348–1.781)	1.058(0.377–3.326)	0.801(0.307–2.086)
Hukou	Agricultural	1.000	1.000	1.000	1.000	1.000	1.000
	Non-agricultural	1.576(1.192–2.083)*	1.295(0.840–1.996)	1.314(0.940–1.839)	1.539(0.825–2.870)	1.086(0.432–2.730)	1.471(0.748–2.894)
Marriage status	Married	1.000	1.000	1.000	1.000	1.000	1.000
	Unmarried	1.554(0.966–2.498)	0.889(0.510–1.548)	1.012(0.653–1.570)	1.430(0.642–3.186)	0.690(0.196–2.432)	0.990(0.414–2.365)
Constant term		0.115(0.055–0.242)*	0.241(0.100–0.548)*	0.277(0.144–0.533)*	0.166(0.044–0.635)	0.312(0.043–1.788)	0.207(0.053–0.805)

Note *$p < 0.05$, RRR: relative-risk ratio, CI: confidence interval

Table 4 Influence of migrant direction and medical insurance on reimbursement ratio

Variables		All samples	West-East	West-Central	West-West
		β(SE)	β(SE)	β(SE)	β(SE)
Migration direction	West-East	0	–	–	–
	West-Central	0.004(0.012)	–	–	–
	West-West	0.041(0.011)*	–	–	–
Medical insurance	NCMS	0	0	0	0
	UEBMI	0.268(0.013)*	0.274(0.018)*	0.252(0.030)*	0.250(0.024)*
	URBMI	0.043(0.017)*	0.070(0.033)*	0.059(0.031)	0.014(0.026)
Residence	Resident committee	0	0	0	0
	Village committee	0.018(0.010)	−0.044(0.016)*	−0.005(0.023)	0.017(0.017)
Gender	Male	0	0	0	0
	Female	0.003(0.011)	−0.020(0.020)	−0.013(0.022)	0.028(0.018)
Age		0.003(0.001)*	0.003(0.001)*	0.002(0.001)	0.003(0.001)*
Race	Han nationality	0	0	0	0
	Minority	0.034(0.016)*	0.030(0.031)	0.066(0.047)	0.030(0.019)
Education	Primary school or below	0	0	0	0
	Junior high school	0.027(0.014)	0.046(0.026)	0.035(0.030)	0.008(0.021)
	Senior high school	0.035(0.017)*	0.051(0.030)	0.059(0.033)	0.006(0.026)
	College or above	0.047(0.019)*	0.098(0.032)*	0.011(0.041)	−0.008(0.030)
Hukou	Agricultural	0	0	0	0
	Non-agricultural	−0.018(0.014)	−0.030(0.023)	−0.026(0.030)	0.012(0.024)
Marriage status	Married	0	0	0	0
	Unmarried	−0.027(0.021)	−0.055(0.036)	0.040(0.038)	−0.032(0.032)
Constant term		0.066(0.031)*	0.062(0.055)	0.11(0.060)	0.102(0.047)*
Sample size		5060	2200	1114	1746

Note *$p < 0.05$, β: coefficient, SE: standard error

NCMS, and it was 0.070 unit higher in migrants with URBMI than in migrants with NCMS ($p < 0.05$). Among internal migrants from the west to the west, the average medical insurance reimbursement ratio in internal migrants with UEBMI was 0.250 unit ($p < 0.05$) higher than that in migrants with NCMS.

4 Discussion

In this chapter, we explore the association between migration direction, medical insurance and health seeking behaviors in Chinese internal migrants, using multinomial logistic regression and multiple linear regression models. The results show that internal migrants from the west to the central and the west were more willing to hospitalized in prefecture-level or above public hospitals, compared with those from the west to the east. Moreover, internal migrants from the west to the west with UEBMI were more likely to go to the public hospitals at the prefecture-level or above. In addition, the reimbursement ratio of internal migrants from the west to the central and west was higher than those from the west to the east. Furthermore, the reimbursement ratio in internal migrants who had URBMI was higher than that in migrants who had NCMS only in the east.

There are several reasons to explain the association with migration direction/medical insurance and health seeking behaviors among internal migrants. Firstly, although there are more medical resources and high-quality health resources in eastern cities with good economic development (Song et al., 2019), it also means more expensive medical expenses in eastern cities. Internal migrants who migrate to eastern cities are more inclined to public hospitals at the county/district level or below than those migrating to central and western cities, as this can reduce the cost of hospitalization. Peng found that the high cost of health service was a significant obstacle to health-care access for 40.5% migrant workers with sickness (Peng, Chang, Zhou, Hu, & Liang, 2010). In addition, previous studies discovered that outpatient visits among residents with diabetes mellitus and hypertensive living in western regions were higher than those in eastern areas (Jin, Zhu, Yuan, & Meng, 2017; Song & Zhang, 2019), which may be caused by the high hospital costs in the eastern region.

Secondly, patients generally seek health care at high-level hospitals in China (Jin et al., 2019). One important reason is the high quality treatment in high-level hospitals. In the central and western regions, medical resources are not enough and medical conditions are poor. Therefore, internal migrants living in the western and central regions have more trust in prefecture-level hospitals, and the first choice for hospitalization is large hospitals. Liu found that patients placed most importance on equipment, medical skill, facility size and travel time (Liu, Kong, Wang, Zhong, & van de Klundert, 2019).

Thirdly, medical insurance affected patients' choice of medical institutions to a certain extent (Du, Han, Fu, & Xie, 2018). Medical insurance is mainly aimed at the population in public hospitals, and the reimbursement ratio of UEBMI is much higher than that of NCMS. Our study found that the reimbursement ratio of UEBMI and URBMI was larger than that of NCMS, which is consistent with the current medical insurance system in China (Han & Meng, 2019). Therefore, internal migrants with UEBMI are more inclined to be hospitalized in the prefecture-level or above public hospitals than those with NCMS. In the analysis on the regional disparities, this hypothesis was further supported in the West-West migrant population, and the reimbursement ratio of migrants with URBMI was higher than those with NCMS within the West-East subgroup. The system of URBMI in the eastern developed regions is relatively perfect. Studies showed that the distribution of health resources in eastern regions was the most equitable, followed by the central regions, and it was the least equitable in the western regions (Zhang et al., 2017). Some studies found that the "regional separation" in the current medical insurance system constituted an institutional barrier to the utilization of health services for internal migrants (Meng & Han, 2019). This shows that the fairness of the medical insurance system still needs to be further improved to fundamentally realize the equalization and accessibility of health services.

In addition, this study found that internal migrants with more education and non-agricultural *hukou* were more likely to be hospitalized in public hospitals at prefecture-level or above, which was consistent with some previous studies (Yin, Xu, & Zheng, 2017). Internal migrants with more education had a higher reimbursement ratio of medical insurance, but in the subgroup analysis, this effect was only significant in the West-East migrant population. This may be due to the complicated medical insurance reimbursement procedures caused by long-distance mobility from the west to the east, and well-educated people are more likely to obtain a higher reimbursement ratio. With the increase of age, the reimbursement ratio of medical insurance showed an increasing trend. The elderly is more likely to suffer from serious diseases, which have a higher level of medical insurance reimbursement (Zhou & Liu, 2016).

There are some limitations to this study. First, this study only considered the internal migrants who migrate from the west to the east, the central and the west because of a small sample size. Second, this study focused on the analysis of UEBMI, URBMI and NCMS. We did not consider other kinds of commercial insurance, which may affect the choice of hospitalization and reimbursement ratio. Third, the reimbursement ratio is calculated based on the hospitalization expenses and reimbursement expenses self-reported, which may exist a recall bias. Fourth, this is a cross-sectional study, and the relationships should not be explained as causal relationships.

Despite these limitations, some innovation should be noted in this study. Many prior literatures used the Anderson health service utilization models to study health seeking behaviors, or to explore the impact of social integration and medical insurance on the health seeking behaviors of migrants. Considering the migration characteristics, especially the migration direction, and exploring the influence of medical insurance on health seeking behaviors among internal migrants are major innovations of this study, which makes the research results more targeted and comprehensive.

5 Conclusion

This study finds that migration directions affect the hospitalization choices and reimbursement ratio of internal migrants. In addition, different medical insurances have different migrant hospitalization choices and reimbursement ratio within different migration directions. Internal migrants from the west to the central and the west are more likely to choose prefecture-level or above public hospitals, and internal migrants from the west to the east have the highest reimbursement ratio for UEBMI. It is recommended that employers in the central and western regions should increase the coverage of reimbursement and insurance costs for UEBMI. Eastern China should carry out subsidies or preferential policies of medical treatment for internal migrants to guide their health seeking behaviors.

References

Christian, B., Young, D., Gibbs, L., de Silva, A., Gold, L., Riggs, E., et al. (2015). Exploring child dental service use among migrant families in metropolitan Melbourne, Australia. *Journal Australian Dental Journal, 60*(2), 200–204.

Colón-Burgos, J. F., Colón-Jordan, H. M., Reyes-Ortiz, V. E., Marin-Centeno, H. A., & Rios-Mota, R. (2014). Disparities and barriers encountered by immigrant dominican mothers accessing prenatal care services in Puerto Rico. *Journal of Immigrant and Minority Health/Center for Minority Public Health, 16*(4), 646–651.

Du, B., Han, X., Fu, L., & Xie, Y. (2018). Health service demand, supply, utilization and health promotion stratiogy selection of the floating population-based on the behavior model of medical service utilization. *Chinese Health Policy Research, 11*(02), 23–29.

Guo, F., Wang, Z., Yang, N., Guo, W., & Li, D. (2008). Medical treatment of infectious diseases among migrant population in Shijingshan District, Beijing. *Capital Journal of Public Health, 2*(2), 72–73.

Guo, J., Zhou, Q., Weng, H., & Wu, Y. (2015). Multi-level logistic regression model analysis of health service utilization and influencing factors of migrant population. *Chinese Health Economics, 34*(03), 50–52.

Han, J., & Meng, Y. (2019). Institutional differences and geographical disparity: the impact of medical insurance on the equity of health services utilization by the floating elderly population - evidence from China. *International Journal for Equity in Health, 18,* 14.

Hong, Y., Li, X., Stanton, B., Lin, D., Fang, X., Rong, M., & Wang, J. (2006). Too costly to be ill: Healthcare access and health-seeking behaviours among rural-to-urban migrants in China. *World health & Population, 8*(2), 22–34.

Huang, J., Chen, Y., & Pong, R. W. (2015). Factors influencing prenatal screening for down's syndrome: Evidence from Zhejiang (China). *Asia-Pacific Journal of Public Health, 27*(2), 1288–1297.

Jiang, H. (2016). A study on the utilization of medical insurance and medical services for the migrant population based on the national mobile population dynamic monitoring data. *The World of Survey and Research, 07,* 14–20.

Jin, Y., Yuan, B., Zhu, W., Zhang, Y., Xu, L., & Meng, Q. (2019). The interaction effect of health insurance reimbursement and health workforce on health care-seeking behaviour in China. *International Journal of Health Planning and Management, 34*(3), 900–911.

Jin, Y., Zhu, W., Yuan, B., & Meng, Q. (2017). Impact of health workforce availability on health care seeking behavior of patients with diabetes mellitus in China. *International Journal for Equity in Health, 16,* 10.

Lam, K. K. F., & Johnston, J. M. (2012). Health insurance and healthcare utilisation for Shenzhen residents: A tale of registrants and migrants? *Bmc Public Health, 12.*

Li, C., Gu, Y., Huang, W., Lv, J., & Zhang, Z. (2010). Study on health service utilization and influencing factors of urban migrant population. *Chinese Primary Health Care, 24*(12), 1–3.

Liu, Y. (2002). Reforming China's urban health insurance system. *Health Policy, 60*(2).

Liu, J. (2011). The present situation and countermeasures of the community medical and health service for migrant workers. *Chinese Journal of Hospital Administration, 27*(2), 135–137.

Liu, S., Hu, C. X., & Mak, S. (2013). Comparison of health status and health care services utilization between migrants and natives of the same ethnic origin-the case of Hong Kong. *International Journal of Environmental Research and Public Health, 10*(2), 606–622.

Liu, Y., Kong, Q., Wang, S., Zhong, L., & van de Klundert, J. (2019). The impact of hospital attributes on patient choice for first visit: Evidence from a discrete choice experiment in Shanghai, China. *Health Policy and Planning*, 1–12.

Liu, C., & Wu, M. (2012). A study on the influence of social relations of rural migrant population in Beijing on their outpatient care behavior. *Chinese Journal of Social Medicine, 29*(2), 112–114.

Ma, Y., Chen, T., & Shi, Q. (2018). Population mobility: Regional differences in employment and income. *Issues in Agricultural Economy* (05), 80–91.

Meng, Y., & Han, J. (2019). Impact of the medical insurance system on the utilization of health services for the migrant population. *Chinese Journal of Population Science* (05), 110–120 + 128.

Meng, Q., Xu, L., Zhang, Y., Qian, J., Cai, M., Xin, Y., Gao, J., Xu, K., Boerma, J. T., & Barber, S. L. (2012). Trends in access to health services and financial protection in China between 2003 and 2011: A cross-sectional study. *Lancet, 379*(9818), 805–814.

Mou, J., Cheng, J., Zhang, D., Jiang, H., Lin, L., & Griffiths, S. M. (2009). Health care utilisation amongst Shenzhen migrant workers: Does being insured make a difference? *Bmc Health Services Research, 9*(1), 214–210.

Peng, Y., Chang, W., Zhou, H., Hu, H., & Liang, W. (2010). Factors associated with health-seeking behavior among migrant workers in Beijing, China. *Bmc Health Services Research, 10,* 10.

Saunders, C. L., Steventon, A., Janta, B., Stafford, M., Sinnott, C., Allen, L., & Deeny, S. R. (2020). Healthcare utilization among migrants to the UK: Cross-sectional analysis of two national surveys. *Journal of health services research & policy*, *0*(0) 1–8.

Shen, Y., Shi, Y., Wang, H., & Sun, B. (2019). A study on the influence of access to medical facilities on patient's access to medical care: An empirical study based on the survey of patients in Shanghai Hospital. *Urban Development Studies, 26*(12), 46–52 + 61.

Song, S., Yuan, B., Zhang, L., Cheng, G., Zhu, W., Hou, Z., & Meng, Q. (2019). Increased inequalities in health resource and access to health care in rural China. *International Journal of Environmental Research and Public Health, 16*(1).

Song, Y., & Zhang, G. (2019). The Utilization of Public Health Service for People with Chronic Diseases in China and Its Influencing Factors. *Chinese Journal of Public Health*, 1–5.

Sun, J., Deng, S., Xiong, X., & Tang, S. (2014). Equity in access to healthcare among the urban elderly in China: Does health insurance matter? *The International Journal of Health Planning and Management, 29*(2), e127–e144.

Tang, Y., Li, Q., He, T., & Zhang, Q. (2016). Research Progress and Enlightenment on Medical Treatment Behavior of China's Migrant Population. *Chinese Journal of Social Medicine, 33*(5), 435–437,438.

Ye, C., Duan, S., Wu, Y., Hu, H., Liu, X., You, H., W, L., Bogg, L., & Dong, H. (2013). A preliminary analysis of the effect of the new rural cooperative medical scheme on inpatient care at a county hospital. *Bmc Health Services Research, 13,* 8.

Yin, Q., Xu, Q., & Zheng, Y. (2017). Analysis on the utilization status and influencing factors of inpatient medical service in floating population. *Chinese Journal of Public Health, 33*(03), 448–451.

Yu, L., & Zhu, Y. (2018). Impact of residential segregation on the health of the migrant population: an analysis-based on data from The National Internal Migrants Dynamic Monitoring Survey of 2014. *Shandong Social Sciences* (06), 120–128.

Zhai, Z., Wang, Y., & Shi, Q. (2019). Where is China's migrant population heading? *Population Research, 43*(02), 6–11.

Zhang, T., Xu, Y., Ren, J., Sun, L., & Liu, C. (2017). Inequality in the distribution of health resources and health services in China: Hospitals versus primary care institutions. *International Journal for Equity in Health, 16*(1), 42–42.

Zhou, Q., & Liu, G. (2016). Household registration differences in health insurance benefits—Based on the study of local and migrant population. *Nankai Economic Studies, 01*, 77–94.

Chapter 4
Minimum Wage Standard and Migrants' Social Health Insurance Take-Up in China

Shengfeng Lu and Sixia Chen

1 Introduction

Recent years have witnessed a growing body of literatures in exploring ways of improving migrants' health conditions. Better health helps migrants to accommodate to the local environment more easily. Furthermore, improving migrants' health helps the government to maintain social integration and stability. Among various policy tools, social health insurance has been regarded effective in reducing health risks and providing health security. However, we find a substantial proportion of migrants not covered by local social security net in China. So why do some eligible people choose not to be insured? Pioneering studies have provided several interesting explanations. Some studies have found that people usually pay less attention to their health conditions when their income increases (Ruhm, 2000). Another strand of literatures have examined the take-up elasticity of social insurance programs and found negative take-up elasticity of insurance premium deductibility, indicating that the low social awareness, choice complexity and a lack of health insurance literacy are important factors leading to the incomplete social insurance take-up (Heim & Lurie, 2009, 2010; Moriya & Simon, 2016). In addition, some studies focus on social health insurance issues in different countries, such as the United States (Sloan & Conover, 1998; Monheit et al., 2001; Baker et al., 2006; Buchmueller & Ohri, 2006; Gould & Hertel-Fernandez, 2010), Turkey (Erus et al., 2015), Indonesia (Sparrow, 2013; Anggriani, et al., 2020), South Korean (Oh & Jeong, 2017), Nepal (Ko et al., 2018), Nigeria (Dokunmu, et al., 2018), and so on; most of them have observed similar results.

S. Lu (✉)
Economics and Management School, Wuhan University, Wuhan, China
e-mail: shengflu@whu.edu.cn

S. Chen
School of Public Finance and Taxation, Zhongnan University of Economics and Law, Wuhan, China

P. Wang (ed.), *The Health Status of Internal Migrants in China*,
https://doi.org/10.1007/978-981-15-4415-6_4

However, few studies investigate the underlying causes for the incomplete social medical insurance take-up in China. This paper tries to add to relevant literature by exploring the relationship between minimum wage standard and migrants' social health insurance enrollment in China. The minimum wage standard policy is applicable to wage and salary workers, and it is one of the most important policies to guarantee people's basic living and encourage people to participate in social welfare programs. This study helps us answer the crucial question of whether income level is a determinant of migrants' social health insurance take-up decision. Moreover, the present study helps us to examine whether a "trade-off" relationship exists between two different social security programs. Finally, the answer is also important for evaluating the effectiveness of public policies concerning migrants, who are in great need of external financial and social assistance.

In this study, we aim to examine three distinct effects happening when the minimum wage standard is enhanced to impact migrants' social health insurance take-up behavior. The first is the "income effect". Because an increased minimum wage standard finally results in higher-level income, people are then more able to afford health insurance (either social or business). Prior studies have provided the evidence of a positive association between income level and health insurance take-up rate. For example, DeLeire et al. (DeLeire, Chappel, Finegold, & Gee, 2017) examined the effect of an insurance cost-sharing reduction reform and found that insurance subsidies were significantly salient to consumers.

The second is known as the "substitution effect". People may have lower willingness to take up social health insurance when they become richer, considering social health insurance is a kind of relatively low-level health security. Some studies (Finn & Goodship, 2014; Bhargava & Manoli, 2015) have documented a negative relationship between incomplete take-up of social benefits and the public policy lowering health insurance cost.

The last one is the "crowd-out" effect. The minimum wage standard is an anti-poverty social security policy tool. When people feel that they have been well protected, their willingness to take up other social programs is more likely to go down. Therefore, whether the minimum wage scheme enhances social health insurance take-up rate depends on which one of the three effects dominates.

Migration within China is mainly driven by low-income rural population who seek to find a higher-paid job in cities. This means that most migrants are very likely to be affected by the minimum wage scheme. The Chinese government officially initiated the minimum wage program in 2003, and the program had rapidly expanded to the whole country within one year. The policy is designed to assure working people that they will be able to afford basic living costs and stay productive. In practice, each provincial (or provincial-level) government has much discretion to determine the minimum wage standard for lower-level governments. For most provinces, the provincial government enhances the wage standard every two or three years. Generally, the provincial government recalculates the minimum wage standard (MWS) for lower-level governments based on four factors: regional economic and fiscal conditions, average market wage and salary, unemployment rate, and urban living expenses. As such, different cities and counties within the same province often have different minimum wage levels. The minimum wage scheme also takes social insurance premium into consideration. In other words, governments subsidize a substantial share of social insurance premium, and they endeavor to make sure that every worker can participate in the social insurance program without financial concerns.

We exploit individual-level data from the China Migrants Dynamic Survey (CMDS) in 2015 and find an empirically negative relationship between minimum wage level and migrants' social medical insurance take-up. We further investigate the underlying mechanisms and find migrants turn to other medical programs which can provide them higher-level health protection when local MWS increases. In addition, they also become less willing to take up any social health insurance as they feel they have been well protected by the minimum wage system. Overall, the "substitution" and "crowd-out" effects both explain the incomplete social health insurance take-up behaviors in China.

This chapter seeks to contribute to the relevant debate in three ways. First and foremost, this paper is among the first to provide estimates of social health insurance/minimum wage gradient from a developing country. Our study provides new evidence on whether the cost reduction of social programs encourages more people to take up social insurance programs. In addition, previous studies seldom examine the "crowd-out" and "substitution" effects between social health insurance program and other social security programs, while this study fills the gap.

Second, this chapter uses a representative health survey of Chinese internal migrants (i.e., migrants within the country). Using this dataset, we are able to estimate important social health insurance take-up gradients and analyze social program take-up behaviors in China's migrants. As migrants' health conditions have an important bearing on social well-being, our study is conducive to devising policies to address social insurance take-up problems for migrants.

Finally, this chapter puts new emphasis on the heterogeneous effects of minimum wage scheme. We find migrants with specific characteristics respond differently to minimum wage changes. These findings have important policy implications and help us improve social insurance scheme properly.

2 Data and Empirical Framework

2.1 Data and Descriptive Statistics

2.1.1 Minimum Wage Standard

We hand-collect the information on minimum wage standards at the city/county level province by province. The minimum wage standard of each province is announced by the provincial human resources and social security department through its official government website. Specifically, the province divides its respective cities and counties into several classes. Each class applies to its specific minimum wage level.

Table 1 MWS for China's three geographical regions (Chinese Yuan (CNY) per month)

Years	Eastern	Central	Western	The lowest	The highest
2003	429	324	340	235 (Jiangxi)	570 (Shanghai)
2004	503	364	412	293 (Shanxi)	635 (Shanghai)
2005	531	399	428	306 (Heilongjiang)	690 (Shanghai)
2006	615	477	521	356 (Ningxia)	750 (Shanghai)
2007	655	517	588	386 (Gansu)	840 (Shanghai)
2008	741	549	661	477 (Hubei)	960 (Shanghai)
2009	741	580	660	507 (Anhui)	960 (Shanghai)
2010	868	727	828	569 (Gansu)	1120 (Shanghai)
2011	1027	799	957	665 (Jiangxi)	1280 (Shanghai)
2012	1120	962	1105	782 (Anhui)	1450 (Shanghai)
2013	1294	1122	1274	900 (Qinghai)	1620 (Shanghai)
2014	1386	1141	1392	995 (Anhui)	1820 (Shanghai)

Note Eastern China includes 11 provinces, i.e., Beijing, Tianjin, Hebei, Liaoning, Shanghai, Jiangsu, Zhejiang, Fujian, Shandong, Guangdong, Hainan. Central China includes 8 provinces, i.e., Shanxi, Jinlin, Heilongjiang, Anhui, Jiangxi, Hennan, Hubei, Hunan. Western China includes 11 provinces, i.e., Inner Mogolia, Guangxi, Chongqing, Sichuan, Guizhou, Yunan, Shaanxi, Gansu, Ningxia, Qinghai, Xinjiang.

This institutional setting provides us a rich variation in MWS changes in different areas and over time.

Table 1 presents the average MWS for three geographical regions of China-eastern, central and western China respectively year by year (Tibet is excluded due to its poor data quality). We calculated each province's MWS by averaging the minimum wage standards implemented by different areas within its jurisdiction.

As shown in Table 1, we find the average MWS of all three regions increases year by year. The eastern provinces have the highest minimum wage level, which is consistent with their economic conditions and high-level living standard. The western provinces come second while the central provinces have the lowest minimum wage level. With respect to provinces, Shanghai (provincial-level) has higher minimum wage level than the rest 29 provinces over the whole sample period.

2.1.2 Introduction to CMDS 2015

The other data set we use in this study is CMDS 2015, which is conducted by the National Health and Family Commission of China. CMDS is conducted in May every year. As respondents are randomly selected each time, we cannot have panel data that allows us to control individual- and year-fixed effects. Therefore, we use the survey data for migrants as cross-sectional data. We choose CMDS 2015 because it provides us the latest health and economic information of China's migrant population. Finally, we have 206,000 observations in total.

The data provides very detailed host area information about the respondent (i.e., information about the county or urban district the respondent lives in), as well as the exact year when the migrant moved into present residence. As a result, we are able to measure the number of years for which each migrant has resided in a locality. Accordingly, we can calculate how much the minimum wage line has been increased since the migrant moved into the host county. We see the MWS increases as an exogenous shock to migrant's income and social security conditions. The MWS variable is measured as the gap between the minimum wage line of host locality in 2014 and the minimum wage line of host locality in the year when the respondent moved in. We use the 2014 minimum wage line as the latest minimum wage standard because the survey was conducted in May, 2015 and respondents reported their conditions in the past year as part of their answers to many questions. In addition, it also gives us a time lag to estimate the effect of minimum wage standard.

However, the data are only reported to the province to which the migrant's household registration (*hukou*) belongs, while excluding the years for which each respondent lives in his (her) *hukou* province, so we cannot measure the extent to which the MWS has increased in respondent's home place. In the empirical analysis, we do not have much concern about MWS changes before the respondent's migration. However, we still control for a full set of *hukou* province dummies to reduce potential estimation biases caused by the absence of controlled MWS increases before migration.

The survey also involves migrants' insurance enrollment status for four kinds of major social health insurance: the New Rural Cooperative Medical Insurance (NRCMI), the Urban Residence Cooperative Medical Insurance (URCMI), the Urban Employee Basic Medical Insurance (UEBMI) and the Urban and Rural Medical Insurance (URMI). The survey also asks the respondent the place where he (she) takes up the specific insurance (local or home). Therefore, we construct four variables to measure migrants' insurance enrollment status. The first one is a dummy variable (insurance_1) indicating whether the migrant participates in any of the four social health insurances (1 = yes, 0 = no). The second variable (insurance_2) measures the number of social health insurances that the respondent takes up. The third (insurance_home) and the fourth (insurance_local) variables provide the information about migrants' insurance enrollment places. Specifically, the insurance_home variable measures whether the migrant has enrolled in social health insurance programs in his (her) *hukou* province, while the insurance_local measures whether the migrant has enrolled in social health insurance programs in the host area.

We have also constructed several control variables. They include gender (1 = male, 0 = female), age, ethnicity (1 = *Han*, 0 = minority), education (1 = primary school or below, 2 = junior high school, 3 = senior high school, 4 = college or above), marital status (1 = not married, 0 = married), number of children, and household registration (1 = non-agricultural *hukou*, 0 = agricultural *hukou*).

Descriptive statistics of variables we use for estimation are presented in Table 2. As shown in Table 2, about 93% of the migrant population takes up social health insurance programs. The *hukou* province's social insurance enrollment rate is 67.2% while local social health insurance take-up rate is much lower (2.9%). A majority of

Table 2 Summary statistics for dependent and independent variables (n = 206,000)

Variables	Mean	SD	Min	Max
Insurance_1	0.933	0.249	0	1
Insurance_2	0.959	0.310	0	2
Insurance_home	0.672	0.470	0	1
Insurance_local	0.029	0.168	0	1
NRCMI	0.683	0.465	0	1
URCMI	0.042	0.201	0	1
UEBMI	0.180	0.385	0	1
URMI	0.058	0.234	0	1
MWS	212.035	342.439	0	1250
Gender	0.531	0.499	0	1
Age	34.775	10.650	15	95
Ethnicity	0.921	0.269	0	1
Education	2.316	0.879	1	4
Marital status	0.211	0.408	0	1
Children number	1.390	0.724	0	9
Hukou	0.164	0.370	0	1

Note SD: standard deviation

migrants choose to take up the NRCMI program, which is consistent with the fact that migrants mainly come from rural areas (1–16.4% = 83.6%). The NRCMI program guarantees rural people's fundamental medical service demand. With respect to the three social programs designed for urban residents, the UEBMI program has the highest take-up rate among migrants (18.0%) while the URCMI has the lowest rate (4.2%).

The sample is quite gender-balanced where male respondents make up 53.1% of the sample and female respondents make up 46.9%. The average age of the sample population is nearly 35 years old. It is reasonable to assume that the majority of our sample individuals work and they are affected by the minimum wage scheme. On average, migrants have received middle school education, give birth to at least one child and most of them are Han people. Finally, only 21.1% of the respondents are not married (single, divorced or widowed) at the time of survey, nearly 80.0% migrants are married.

2.2 Empirical Analytical Frameworks

In our study, we examine the empirical relationship between minimum wage increases and migrant health insurance take-up behavior. Specifically, we estimate a linear model that is specified as follows:

$$insurance_i = \alpha + \beta MWSL_i + \gamma X_i + \sum \lambda_p + \varepsilon_i \tag{1}$$

where β is the focus of our interest, measuring the association between the minimum wage and migrant's insurance take-up status, X_i represents full sets of individual and household controls. λ_p represents a set of provincial-level dummies, which control for time-invariant unobserved home province characteristics that impact migrants' social health insurance take-up willingness.

The OLS methodologys is used for model estimation. We also exploit the probit model to estimate the model for robustness. However, no matter which methodology we use, the cross-sectional data precludes us from controlling panel fixed effects. The most serious econometric issue of the estimation is omitted bias, which will make migration decision endogenously determined. To be more specific, once the decision of where and when to migrate is endogenously made, the extent to which migrants are affected by the minimum wage scheme is endogenously determined. We adopt two ways to ease omitted bias concern. We first control a set of host city dummies, considering that migrants choose migration destination conditional on economic and social characteristics of the host area. Then, we include a variable denoting each migrant's residence year since he (she) moves into present living place (res_year). The longer the migrant lives in the host area, the larger extent to which the migrant is affected by local MWS changes. With the inclusion of such a variable, we are able to mitigate the estimation bias caused by the migrant's purposely choosing the migration year.

3 Empirical Analysis

3.1 *Minimum Wage Increase and Migrant's Social Health Insurance Participation*

Our regressions start with a variety of individual controls. The explanatory variables in model specification (1) in Table 3 include: gender, age, ethnicity, education, marital status, children number. In specifications (2) and (3), we continue to include home province dummies and host city dummies in the estimation model, respectively. Standard errors are clustered at the city level. The regression results are presented in specifications (1)–(3) in Table 3.

We find a significantly negative relationship between MWS and migrants' social health insurance take-up status, especially after we control province and city dummies. A significantly negative relationship between MWS and the number of social health insurances is also expected. On average, the minimum wage increases by 1200 CNY (i.e., 100 CNY per month), the likelihood of the migrant taking up social insurance decreases by 1.56% of a standard deviation.

We are concerned that estimates from specifications (1)–(3) can be biased by omitted variables. For instance, the longer migrants live in their host areas, the more

Table 3 MWS and migrants' social insurance take-up status

Variables	Specification (1)		Specification (2)		Specification (3)		Specification (4)		Specification (5)	
	Insurance_1	Insurance_2	Insurance_1	Insurance_2	Insurance_1	Insurance_2	Insurance_1	Insurance_2	Insurance_1	Insurance_2
MWS	−0.000016 (−1.58)	−0.000028*** (−4.20)	−0.000012 (−1.35)	−0.000025*** (−4.17)	−0.000014** (−2.35)	−0.000013*** (−2.65)	−0.000014** (−2.27)	−0.00001** (−2.11)	−0.000015** (−2.47)	−0.000014*** (−2.80)
Gender	0.0155*** (6.71)	0.0087*** (6.47)	0.0140*** (6.23)	0.0076*** (5.73)	0.0144*** (6.29)	0.0075*** (5.78)	0.0146*** (6.62)	0.0082*** (6.27)	0.0141*** (6.19)	0.0081*** (6.22)
Age	−0.0006*** (−3.10)	0.0001 (1.10)	−0.0001 (−0.59)	0.0005*** (4.60)	−0.0001 (−0.67)	0.0003*** (2.68)	−0.0001 (−0.41)	0.0004*** (3.67)	−0.0001 (−0.38)	0.0003*** (3.01)
Ethnicity	0.0112 (1.50)	0.0080 (1.40)	0.0025 (0.45)	0.0060 (1.34)	0.00005 (0.01)	0.0033 (0.85)	0.0001 (0.02)	0.0034 (0.88)	−0.0002 (−0.03)	0.0031 (0.79)
Education	0.0087*** (5.11)	0.0053*** (2.98)	0.0093*** (5.83)	0.0057*** (3.39)	0.0050*** (3.13)	0.0031 (1.64)	0.0050*** (3.10)	0.0030 (1.59)	0.0045** (2.84)	0.0026 (1.42)
Marital status	−0.0451*** (−6.63)	−0.0405*** (−6.70)	−0.0396*** (−6.15)	−0.0363*** (−6.34)	−0.0401*** (−6.33)	−0.0383*** (−7.09)	−0.0402*** (−6.35)	−0.0386*** (−7.13)	−0.0392*** (−6.15)	−0.0374*** (−6.89)
Children number	0.0102*** (4.48)	0.0060*** (3.23)	0.0016 (1.19)	−0.0001 (−0.10)	0.0018 (1.40)	0.0002 (0.20)	0.0019 (1.54)	0.0006 (0.62)	0.0019 (1.45)	0.0003 (0.28)
Res_year							−0.0002 (−0.78)	−0.0006*** (−3.75)		
Nutrition									−0.0050* (−1.88)	−0.0066*** (−3.10)
Family planning									−0.0064** (−2.36)	−0.0065*** (−2.92)
Smoking									−0.0094*** (−3.68)	−0.0041** (−2.08)
Constant	0.9387*** (77.01)	0.9068*** (89.00)	0.7835*** (14.61)	0.7735*** (14.25)	0.7945*** (14.39)	0.8000*** (14.42)	0.7947*** (14.38)	0.8122*** (14.98)	0.8193*** (14.86)	0.8308*** (15.43)
Province dummies	No	No	Yes	Yes	Yes	Yes	Yes	Yes	Yes	Yes
City dummies	No	No	No	No	Yes	Yes	Yes	Yes	Yes	Yes

(continued)

Table 3 (continued)

Variables	Specification (1)		Specification (2)		Specification (3)		Specification (4)		Specification (5)	
	Insurance_1	Insurance_2	Insurance_1	Insurance_2	Insurance_1	Insurance_2	Insurance_1	Insurance_2	Insurance_1	Insurance_2
R^2	0.0031	0.0032	0.0134	0.0136	0.0376	0.0345	0.0376	0.0347	0.0381	0.0350
n	157,167	159,191	157,167	159,191	157,167	159,191	157,167	159,191	157,167	159,191

Variables	Specification (6)						Specification (7)			
	Insurance_home	Insurance_local	Insurance_home	Insurance_local	Insurance_home	Insurance_local	Insurance_home	Insurance_local	Insurance_home	Insurance_local
MWS	−0.00013*** (−7.69)	0.000012** (2.37)	−0.00012*** (−6.88)	0.0000122*** (2.79)	−0.000082*** (−7.76)	0.0000126*** (3.02)	−0.000073*** (−7.50)	0.000012*** (2.92)	−0.00008*** (−7.78)	0.0000127*** (3.03)
Constant	1.1618*** (36.86)	0.0437*** (5.61)	0.9011*** (14.67)	0.0497 (1.62)	0.7807*** (12.79)	0.1138*** (3.97)	0.7828*** (12.69)	0.1136*** (3.96)	0.7701*** (13.03)	0.1075*** (3.77)
Res_year							Yes	Yes		
Nutrition									Yes	Yes
Family planning									Yes	Yes
Smoking									Yes	Yes
Controls	Yes	Yes	Yes	Yes	Yes	Yes	Yes	Yes	Yes	Yes
Province dummies	No	No	Yes	Yes	Yes	Yes	Yes	Yes	Yes	Yes
City dummies	No	No	No	No	Yes	Yes	Yes	Yes	Yes	Yes
R^2	0.1174	0.0032	0.1357	0.0105	0.1860	0.0582	0.1866	0.0614	0.1861	0.0616
n	159,191	159,191	159,191	159,191	159,191	152,655	159,189	159,189	159,191	159,191

Note MWS: minimum wage standard. Standard errors are clustered at the household level; *T* values are reported in brackets; ***, **, * indicate statistical significance at the 1%, 5%, and 10% levels, respectively.

likely migrants are to experience a higher local GDP growth. The higher GDP growth would enhance the minimum wage and change people's willingness to participate in social health insurance programs simultaneously. For another example, migrants are usually low-income and care less about their health conditions, which makes them less willing to take up social health insurance programs. To ameliorate omitted variable bias, we separately include the variable of residence years (res_year) in specification (4), and another three dummies indicating whether the respondent cares about his (her) health conditions in specification (5). The three dummies include whether the respondent has gained any knowledge of nutrition, family planning and smoking control in the last year, respectively (1 = yes, 0 = no).

When the residence year variable and three dummies are respectively included in the estimation, we still find a significantly negative relationship between MWS and social health insurance take-up status, albeit with smaller coefficients. As for the additional controls, residence year does not affect migrant social health insurance take-up status. However, the probability of participating in social health insurance programs decreases as long as the migrant cares more about his (her) health conditions. The results demonstrate a "trade-off" effect between health consciousness and social health insurance participation.

We further examine whether the minimum wage affects the geographical distribution of social health insurance enrollment. Results are explored by alternating dependent variables in specification (3). The results in specifications (6)–(7) show that migrants have lower social health insurance take-up rates in home provinces, but they have a higher level of social insurance enrollment in their host areas. The extent to which migrants increase social health insurance participation in their host areas is smaller than the extent to which migrants social health insurance participation is reduced in their home provinces. Migrants may abandon NRCMI program since they are more protected by the minimum wage scheme. The overall effect of MWS on social insurance is still negative.

Finally, we use the probit model to re-estimate Regression (1). We do not report the results for brevity. However, we still find a statistically negative relationship between MWS and migrants' social insurance take-up rate.

3.2 *Identifying Possible Channels: Income, Employment Status and Social Insurance Enrollment Transmission*

In this subsection, we continue to identify possible channels through which the above relationship exists. We examine three channels: income level, employment status, and social insurance enrollment transmission.

For the first two channels, our identification strategy contains two steps. First, we establish a positive relationship between MWS and the factors that are supposed to affect migrants' social health insurance enrollment. Second, we include those factors in the estimation model and record how the coefficients of the MWS variable change

Table 4 Minimum wage increases and channel factors

Channel	Household income	Household income	Employment	Employment
MWS	1.2414*** (4.35)	0.9077*** (3.64)	0.0000 (0.52)	0.000033*** (5.46)
Constant	7009.581*** (7.13)	5607.358*** (2.91)	0.7963*** (14.93)	0.5780*** (8.96)
Control variables	No	Yes	No	Yes
Province dummies	Yes	Yes	Yes	Yes
City dummies	Yes	Yes	Yes	Yes
R^2	0.0472	0.0637	0.0632	0.1384
n	200,207	159,191	200,207	159,191

Note MWS: minimum wage standard. Standard errors are clustered at the household level; *T* values are reported in brackets; ***, **, * indicate statistical significance at the 1%, 5%, and 10% levels, respectively.

with that inclusion. If the significantly negative effect is reduced in the estimation, our examination suggests that the social insurance take-up behavior of migrants is influenced through these two channels.

We use a variable-representing total household income as our first intermediate variable. The second intermediate variable we use is migrants' employment status. It is measured as a binary variable: whether the respondent has a paid-job or not. We examine the relationship between MWS and these two channel factors, and the results are shown in Table 4. We find MWS is positively associated with two channel factors we have considered. On average, migrants who have experienced MWS increases are significantly more likely to have more household income, and they are more likely to be employed as well.

After establishing a positive relationship between MWS and intermediate factors that may affect migrants' social health insurance take-up behavior, we investigate how the relationship between MWS and social health insurance participation changes after these possible channels are controlled for. Table 5 demonstrates the results when two channel factors are added to model specification (3). However, we do not observe a significant reduction in the coefficients of MWS variable after we control these channel factors. Instead, we find that the coefficients of MWS become even larger. The results confirm that neither household income nor employment status significantly affect migrants' social health insurance take-up behavior. In other words, since social health insurance programs are heavily subsidized by the government, income level does not play an important role in affecting people's determination to take up social insurance programs. "Income effect" may be very little in our study.

In order to explore why migrants reduce their social insurance take-up behaviors, we turn to the third explanation: social insurance enrollment transmission. Specifically, we aim to find which social health insurance is increasingly taken up by

Table 5 Possible channels: household income and employment status

Variables	Insurance_1	Insurance_2	Insurance_H	Insurance_L	Insurance_1	Insurance_2	Insurance_H	Insurance_L
MWS	−0.000014** (−2.30)	−0.0000131*** (−2.63)	−0.00008*** (−7.68)	0.0000125*** (3.02)	−0.0000162*** (−2.70)	−0.0000143*** (−2.91)	−0.000081*** (−7.55)	0.0000128*** (3.07)
Household income	−0.0000** (−2.36)	−0.0000 (−1.43)	−0.0000*** (−3.55)	0.0000 (0.51)				
Employ_status					0.0543*** (6.39)	0.0310*** (5.76)	−0.0346*** (−4.84)	−0.00819*** (−3.31)
Constant	0.7966*** (14.35)	0.8125*** (14.95)	0.7891*** (12.94)	0.1135*** (3.96)	0.7635*** (13.38)	0.7936*** (14.38)	0.8006*** (12.69)	0.1185*** (4.14)
Control variables	Yes	Yes	Yes	Yes	Yes	Yes	Yes	Yes
Province dummies	Yes	Yes	Yes	Yes	Yes	Yes	Yes	Yes
City dummies	Yes	Yes	Yes	Yes	Yes	Yes	Yes	Yes
R2	0.0377	0.0345	0.1867	0.0614	0.0415	0.0364	0.1867	0.0617
n	157,167	159,191	159,191	159,191	157,167	159,191	159,191	159,191

Note MWS: minimum wage standard. Standard errors are clustered at the household level; *T* values are reported in brackets; ***, **, * indicate statistical significance at the 1%, 5%, and 10% levels, respectively.

Table 6 Possible channels: social health insurance enrollment transmission

Variables	NRCMI	URCMI	UEBMI	URMI
MWS	−0.00007*** (−6.28)	0.0000** (2.01)	0.0000359*** (4.88)	0.0000141*** (2.69)
constant	0.9530*** (15.27)	−0.0099 (−0.31)	−0.2526*** (−3.16)	0.0542 (0.89)
Control variables	Yes	Yes	Yes	Yes
Province dummies	Yes	Yes	Yes	Yes
City dummies	Yes	Yes	Yes	Yes
R2	0.2337	0.1727	0.2332	0.0701
n	151,746	151,260	151,445	151,333

Note MWS: minimum wage standard. Standard errors are clustered at the household level; *T* values are reported in brackets; ***, **, * indicate statistical significance at the 1%, 5%, and 10% levels, respectively.

migrants and which social insurance is decreasingly taken up. The dependent variable is replaced with the take-up rate of a specific kind of social health insurance. The detailed results are shown in Table 6.

By investigating into the third channel, we find both "substitution" and "crowd out" effects explain the negative relationship between MWS and social health insurance enrollment. On average, the NRCMI take-up rate decreases by 8.4% when the MWS increases by 1200 CNY(100 CNY per month). By contrast, the UEBMI and the URMI's take-up rates increase by 4.3% and 1.69%, respectively. The relationship between MWS and URCMI take-up rate is also significantly positive, but the economic significance is not large enough.

Among the four social health insurance programs, NRCMI requires the lowest insurance premium, but it only provides the lowest health protection. The result, to some degree, confirms the "substitution" effect. To be more specific, people prefer the kind of social health insurance which provides them higher-level medical treatment and health services once they can afford more investment in health. In addition, as the NRCMI program requires participants to enroll in their *hukou* province, the results are also consistent with the fact that fewer migrants enroll in social medical insurance programs at home when they get higher-paid jobs in host areas.

The sum of coefficients of the MWS variable from the NRCMI model to the URMI model is −0.0000197, which is significantly smaller than the coefficient of the MWS variable in specification (3) in Table 3. The unexplained part (−0.0000197–(−0.000013) = −0.0000067) could be possibly due to the "crowd-out" effect. That is, as the minimum wage scheme is a public policy providing social security, people may feel so well protected that they reduce participation in other social insurance programs.

Overall, our channel examinations indicate that the "crowd out" and "substitution" effects dominate when migrants' social health insurance take-up behavior is affected by the minimum wage scheme. The results have important policy implications. We suggest that the NRCMI program which requires people to enroll in their home provinces may be not an effective policy to improve migrants' health protection. A social health insurance that can provide higher-level medical services and facilitate migrants' enrollment in their host areas is more expected. Besides, the government should implement more health education programs to improve migrants' health consciousness.

3.3 Heterogeneous Associations Between MWS and Social Health Insurance Take-up Rate

In this section, we examine how the relationship between MWS and social health insurance take-up rate that is introduced in specification (3) may differ by specific individual characteristics. We conduct four heterogeneity tests, and the results are presented in Table 7.

The first test is to examine the heterogeneous associations between two groups: migrants who are registered as urban residents (non-agricultural *hukou*) and migrants who are registered as rural residents (agricultural *hukou*). We find the negative health insurance take-up behavior is mainly driven by rural migrants. Although urban migrants reduce their insurance take-up rate in their home provinces and increase the take-up rate in their host areas, the net effect is not statistically significant. Rural

Table 7 Heterogeneity tests for the association between MWS and social health insurance take-up

Groups	Insurance_1	Insurance_2	Insurance_H	Insurance_L
Hukou = non-agricultural	−0.000012 (−1.12)	−0.0000135 (−1.33)	−0.0000394*** (−3.43)	0.0000*** (2.83)
Hukou = agricultural	−0.000012* (−1.86)	−0.0000109*** (−2.32)	−0.0000787*** (−6.71)	0.0000124*** (2.66)
Work-oriented migration	−0.000017** (−2.44)	−0.000013** (−2.38)	−0.0000754*** (−6.46)	0.0000104*** (2.61)
Family-oriented migration	0.0000 (0.31)	−0.0000 (−0.67)	−0.0000967*** (−5.51)	0.000024** (2.25)
Moving across province	−0.0000178* (−1.72)	−0.0000142* (−1.68)	−0.0000898*** (−6.49)	0.0000116*** (2.92)
Moving within province	−0.0000 (−1.47)	−0.0000** (−2.13)	−0.0000641*** (−5.54)	0.0000127** (2.09)
Formally employed	−0.0000 (−0.47)	0.0000 (0.47)	−0.00007*** (−3.88)	0.0000* (1.76)
Informally employed	−0.0000133*** (−2.15)	−0.0000125** (−2.55)	−0.00007*** (−6.92)	0.0000126*** (2.85)

Note Standard errors are clustered at the household level; T values are reported in brackets; ***, **, * indicate statistical significance at the 1%, 5%, and 10% levels, respectively migrants are more likely to reduce the social insurance enrollment as well as the number of social health insurance types that they would take up. On average, whenever minimum wage increases by 1200 CNY per year, rural migrants would be 9.44% less likely to enroll in social health insurance plan in their home provinces, while 1.49% more likely to enroll in their host areas. The results imply the overall effect is driven by the rural sub-sample, and this is consistent with the fact that most migrants are rural people.

The second heterogeneity test is related to migration motives. Our survey provides seven causes of why the respondents become migrants: work and business, study and training, the enlistment, settlement with family members, marriage, house demolition and removal, and going to relatives and friends for help. We categorize the first three as work-oriented migration and the last four as family-oriented migration. The first type of migration is more likely to be affected by the minimum wage scheme. The results show that the negative relationship mainly exists among work-oriented migrants. For the family-oriented migrants, the relationship between minimum wage scheme and medical insurance take-up rate is not statistically significant. However, the medical insurance take-up rate of family-oriented migrants decreases in their home provinces and increases in their host areas.

Thirdly, we divide the samples into two types. One type includes migrants who migrate within their home provinces, and the other type includes migrants who migrate across provinces. We do not find significant differences between these two types. For migrants, whether they migrate across provincial borders or not, the MWS always reduces their social health insurance participation.

Finally, we categorize respondents who are employed in public sectors into two groups. We find that the negative association between MWS and social health insurance enrollment mainly exists among migrants who are not formally employed. The formally employed migrants only account for roughly 5.30% of the sample. Their social health insurance enrollment willingness does not significantly change even since minimum wage increases. However, the take-up rate of social health insurance in home provinces for formally employed migrants goes down. On the other hand, we find a statistically negative relationship among informally employed migrants. These migrants are usually low-income people who are most likely to be protected by the minimum wage scheme. After minimum wage increases, their social health insurance enrollment willingness decreases.

4 Conclusions

Social health insurance is supposed to provide basic health services for people who need social assistance when they are sick. However, in recent years, China has failed to realize a full coverage of social health insurance program. In this study, we mainly examine the empirical relationship between minimum wage and migrants' social health insurance participation. Using data from CMDS 2015, we find a statistically significant and negative relationship between minimum wage and migrants' social health insurance taking-up rate. Furthermore, the "substitution" and "crowd-out" effects both give rise to that negative relationship. On one hand, migrants tend to participate in medical programs which can provide them higher-level health protection since the minimum wage increases. On the other hand, migrants' participation in social health programs decreases as long as they feel well protected by other social security programs. Finally, we find migrants with specific characteristics respond differently to minimum wage increases. For example, we find the overall effect is driven by rural sub-sample. For another example, social health program participation by migrants who migrate for work and those who are not formally employed decreases more significantly than that by other migrants when MWS increases.

The present study has some important policy implications. The results indicate a social health insurance that can provide higher-level medical services for poorer people is more expected. The government should implement more health education programs to improve migrants' health consciousness.

References

Anggriani, Y., Ramadaniati, H. U., Sarnianto, P., Pontoan, J., & Suryawati, S. (2020). The impact of pharmaceutical policies on medicine procurement pricing in Indonesia under the implementation of Indonesia's social health insurance system. *Value in Health Regional Issues, 21*, 1–8.

Baker, D., Sudano, J., Durazo-Arvizu, R., Feinglass, J., Witt, W., & Thompson, J. (2006). Health insurance coverage and the risk of decline in overall health and death among the near elderly, 1992–2002. *Medical Care, 44*(3), 277–282.

Bhargava, S., & Manoli, D. (2015). Psychological frictions and the incomplete take-up of social benefits: Evidence from an IRS field experiment. *American Economic Review, 105*(11), 3489–3529.

Buchmueller, T., & Ohri, S. (2006). Health insurance take-up by the near-elderly. *Health Services Research, 41*(6), 2054–2073.

DeLeire, T., Chappel, A., Finegold, K., & Gee, E. (2017). Do individuals respond to cost-sharing subsidies in their selections of marketplace health insurance plans? *Journal of Health Economics, 56*, 71–86.

Dokunmu, T. M., Adjekukor, C. U., Oladejo, D. O., & Amoo, E. O. (2018). Dataset on analysis of quality of health and social insurance subscription in different socio-economic class of workers in selected areas in southwest Nigeria. *Data in Brief, 21*, 1286-1291.

Erus, B., Yakut-Cakar, B., Cali, S., & Adaman, F. (2015). Health policy for the poor: An exploration on the take-up of means-tested health benefits in Turkey. *Social Science & Medicine, 130*, 99-106.

Finn, D., & Goodship, J. (2014). *Take-up of benefits and poverty: An evidence and policy review*. London: Centre for Economic and Social Inclusion.

Gould, E., & Hertel-Fernandez, A. (2010). Early retiree and near-elderly health insurance in recession. *Journal of Aging & Social Policy, 22*(2), 172-187.

Heim, B. T., & Lurie, I. Z. (2009). Do increased premium subsidies affect how much health insurance is purchased? Evidence from the self-employed. *Journal of Health Economics, 28*(6), 1197–1210.

Heim, B. T., & Lurie, I. Z. (2010). The effect of self-employed health insurance subsidies on self-employment. *Journal of Public Economics, 94*(11–12), 995–1007.

Ko, H., Kim, H., Yoon, C., & Kim, C. (2018). Social capital as a key determinant of willingness to join community-based health insurance: A household survey in Nepal, *Public Health, 160*, 52-61.

Monheit, A. C., Vistnes, J. P., & Eisenberg, J. M. (2001). Moving to medicare: Trends in the health insurance status of near-elderly workers, 1987-1996. *Health Affairs, 20*(2), 204-213.

Moriya, A. S., & Simon, K. (2016). Impact of premium subsidies on the take-up of health insurance: Evidence from the 2009 American Recovery and Reinvestment Act (ARRA). *American Journal of Health Economics, 2*(3), 318–343.

Oh, H., & Jeong, C. H., (2017). Korean immigrants don't buy health insurance: The influences of culture on self-employed Korean immigrants focusing on structure and functions of social networks. *Social Science & Medicine, 191*, 194-201.

Ruhm, C. J. (2000). Parental leave and child health. *Journal of Health Economics, 19*(6), 931–960.

Sloan, F. A. & Conover, S. C. J. (1998). Life transitions and health insurance coverage of the near elderly. *Medical Care, 36*(2), 110–125.

Sparrow, R., Suryahadi, A., & Widyanti, W. (2013). Social health insurance for the poor: Targeting and impact of Indonesia's Askeskin programme. *Social Science & Medicine, 96*, 264-271.

Chapter 5
Identity Patterns and the Health of Internal Migrants

Tao Zhong and Junfeng Jiang

1 Introduction

The Constitution of the World Health Organization (WHO) states that health is a state of complete physical, mental and social well-being and not merely the absence of disease or infirmity (Tang & Li, 2019). Health is vital for the growth of social well-being and realization of fairness and justice, which is an inevitable requirement for promoting the all-round development of people. Currently, universal health has been considered as a sign of success of health policies and reforms (Lairson, Hindson, & Hauquitz, 1995). The *Healthy China 2030* was also proposed as a national strategy in 2015.

With the rapid development of urbanization, Chinese internal migrants reached 244 million in 2017 (National Bureau of Statistics, 2018), who have become an important part of employees in China. Migrating into other places, they often face a new working and living environment, and are affected by the dual division household registration system. With a more fragile psychology and exposing to more health risks, they usually have more physical and mental health problems (Chen, Zhang, & Yu, 2018). It is reported that the health level of Chinese internal migrants in the host areas has been declining in recent years (Wang, 2016), which is mainly manifested by the existence of chronic stress (Yu & Yu, 2018). Thus, improving the health of Chinese internal migrants has become an important task of the *Healthy China 2030*.

In recent years, the health of Chinese internal migrants has received more and more attention. Most scholars have studied migrants' health from the perspective of social support (Yan, Peng, Liu, & Zhang, 2009; Yu & Yu, 2018) and social cohesion (Wang & Chen, 2015; Yang, Zhang, & Zhang, 2016), but less frequently from the perspective of identity. Social cohesion is not only the identity of individuals to groups

T. Zhong (✉) · J. Jiang
School of Health Sciences, Wuhan University, Wuhan, China
e-mail: zhongtao327657854@qq.com

P. Wang (ed.), *The Health Status of Internal Migrants in China*,
https://doi.org/10.1007/978-981-15-4415-6_5

and communities but also the acceptance of individuals by communities and groups. Identity is a part of social cohesion, and it is considered a higher level of social cohesion. The social identity theory indicates that sense of belonging to a certain group will strongly influence perceptions, attitudes and behaviors (Tajfel, 1978), which suggests the importance of identity (Fromm, 2001). More sense of belonging to a certain group can bring more happiness (Guo & Xing, 2009), thus positively influencing people's physical and mental health (Bracke, 2001; Hale, Hannum, & Espelage, 2005). Previous studies show that Chinese internal migrants usually lack the sense of belonging to local areas and have difficulties in integration. Thus, they often manifest uncertain, ambiguous and self-contradictory identity (Li & Zhang, 2012; Shi, 2016). One study conducted in children who moved to urban areas shows that an unambiguous identity is related to a better mental health status (Chen et al., 2018). However, some studies show that identity has little or nonsignificant effect on mental health (Shan, 2011). It is found that the impact of identity on health is still inconsistent currently, and the impact of identity patterns on the health of Chinese internal migrants is also less frequently discussed in China. Therefore, this study attempted to examine the association between identity patterns and migrants' physical/mental health to provide scientific evidence for the improvement of their overall health.

2 Data and Method

2.1 Data Source

The data used in this chapter were derived from the Volume C of the China Migrants Dynamic Survey (CMDS) in 2014. This survey included data collected in Beijing, Qingdao, Xiamen, Jiaxing, Shenzhen, Zhongshan, Zhengzhou and Chengdu cities. A stratified, multistage, probability-proportionate-to-size (PPS) sampling method was used. They collected a sample size of n = 15,999 migrants aged 15–59 years who lived in the host areas for at least one month but did not have local *hukou*. The cases with missing values on identity and health indicators were deleted, so the sample size n = 15,997 was used for the analysis.

2.2 Variables and Classification Criteria

General health was measured using the General Health Subscale in SF-36, including six indicators (see Table 1). SF-36 is widely used to evaluate health-related quality of life with satisfactory reliability and validity (Wang et al., 2016; Ware & Gandek, 1998). In this study, the Cronbach α coefficient of the General Health Subscale was 0.834, indicating an acceptable reliability of this scale. The six indicators were added to yield a general health index ranging from 6 to 30, and higher scores meant better general health.

Table 1 Measures of health and identity

	Indicators	Range	α
General health	In general, would you say your health is	1–5 (poor-excellent)	0.834
	Compared to one year ago, how would you rate your health in general now	1–5 (much worse-much better)	
	I seem to get sick a little easier than other people	1–5 (absolutely correct-absolutely wrong)	
	I expect my health to get worse	1–5 (absolutely correct-absolutely wrong)	
	I am as healthy as anybody I know	1–5 (absolutely wrong-absolutely correct)	
	My health is excellent	1–5 (absolutely wrong-absolutely correct)	
Mental health	I feel nervous	1–5 (never-always)	0.782
	I feel despaired	1–5 (never-always)	
	I feel restlessness or irritable	1–5 (never-always)	
	I feel depressed	1–5 (never-always)	
	It's hard for me to work	1–5 (never-always)	
	I feel worthless	1–5 (never-always)	
Identity	I am a part of this city (urban identity)	0–1 (disagree-agree)	
	I feel that the natives are willing to accept me as a member of them (local acceptance)	0–1 (disagree-agree)	
	Do you plan to live locally for a long time (willingness of long-term residence)	0–1 (no-yes)	
	If policy permitted, whether you are willing to move your *hukou* to local areas (willingness of *hukou* moving)	0–1 (no-yes)	

Mental health was measured using the 6-item Kessler Mental Disorder Scale (K6) (see Table 1). The K6 is widely used to assess non-specific mental health problems and mental illnesses in general population, such as stress and anxiety, and is confirmed to have good reliability and validity in China (Xu et al., 2013; Zheng, Xu, Zhou, & Li, 2009). In this study, the Cronbach α coefficient of K6 was 0.782, indicating an acceptable reliability of this scale. The six indicators were added to yield a mental health index ranging from 6 to 30, and higher scores meant better mental health.

Four indicators, including urban identity, local acceptance, willingness of long-term residence and willingness of *hukou* moving, were used as the measures of identity (see Table 1).[1] All four indicators were binary.

Gender, age, ethnicity, *hukou*, marital status, socioeconomic status (SES) (including education, occupational status and personal income) and migration factors (including range/distance and duration of migration) were used as control variables. Prior evidence suggests that there might be a nonlinear relationship between age and subjective health (Jiang & Wang, 2018), so the square of age was also used as a control variable. In order to eliminate the scale effect, the age_squared variable was divided by 100. Details can be seen in Table 2.

2.3 Statistical Methods

Because four identity variables were binary, the latent class analysis (LCA) was used to describe the latent class of identity in Chinese internal migrants. LCA is used to interpret the correlation between observed variables through latent class variables to achieve local independence (Qiu, 2008). Latent Gold version 4.5 software was used for the performance of LCA. Because the sample size was larger than 1000, the Bayesian Information Criterion (BIC) was used to examine the goodness of fit of the model (Lin & Dayton, 1997).

All other analyses were performed using SPSS version 22.0. Univariate analyses, including t test and F test, were used to examine the group disparities in health, and Pearson correlation analysis was used to examine the correlation between health and age/duration of migration. The ordinary least squares (OLS) model was used to examine the influencing factors of general and mental health. $p < 0.05$ was considered statistically significant.

3 Results

3.1 Basic Information

The average age of Chinese internal migrants was 32.08 ± 8.72 years, and the average duration of migration was 4.25 ± 4.43 years. Most internal migrants were Han nationality (96.5%), males (55.0%), married (73.4%), inter-provincial (54.8%), and from rural areas (86.0%). A low SES was observed, only 14.7% of the migrants received higher education, 11.6% of the migrants earned more than 5000 Chinese Yuan (CNY) per month, 63.1% of the migrants were employees, and 9.1% of the migrants did not have a stable job. Most internal migrants believed that they belonged

[1] Identity selection indicator refers Hou's study (Hou & Yao, 2016).

Table 2 Basic information of Chinese internal migrants (N = 15,997)

Variables	n (%)	General health score		Mental health score	
		M ± SD	*t/F*	M ± SD	*t/F*
		23.22 ± 3.87		26.58 ± 3.07	
Gender			7.77***		0.95
Male	8798 (55.0)	23.43 ± 3.84		26.60 ± 3.11	
Female	7199 (45.0)	22.95 ± 3.88		26.55 ± 3.02	
Ethnicity			2.54*		−1.07
Han nationality	15,434 (96.5)	23.23 ± 3.87		26.57 ± 3.08	
Minority	563 (3.5)	22.81 ± 3.88		26.71 ± 2.84	
Marital status			−7.77***		8.77***
Married	11,743 (73.4)	23.08 ± 3.91		26.70 ± 3.05	
Unmarried	4254 (26.6)	23.60 ± 3.73		26.22 ± 3.10	
Hukou			−4.76***		−2.46*
Agricultural	13,757 (86.0)	23.28 ± 3.86		26.60 ± 3.03	
Non-agricultural	2240 (14.0)	22.86 ± 3.90		26.42 ± 3.30	
Range of migration			7.28**		2.48
Inter-provincial	8769 (54.8)	23.13 ± 3.88		26.53 ± 3.15	
Cross-city within province	6635 (41.5)	23.30 ± 3.86		26.62 ± 3.00	
Cross-county within city	593 (3.7)	23.63 ± 3.78		26.75 ± 2.75	
Education			18.29***		15.22***
Primary school or below	1504 (9.4)	22.72 ± 4.02		26.70 ± 3.02	
Junior high school	8084 (50.5)	23.33 ± 3.84		26.71 ± 2.98	
Senior high school	4051 (25.3)	23.37 ± 3.84		26.40 ± 3.18	
College or above	2358 (14.7)	22.89 ± 3.86		26.34 ± 3.19	

(continued)

Table 2 (continued)

Variables	n (%)	General health score		Mental health score	
		M ± SD	*t/F*	M ± SD	*t/F*
Personal income monthly (CNY)			3.63*		4.85**
Less than 3000	6499 (40.6)	23.12 ± 3.91		26.53 ± 3.07	
3000 to 5000	7640 (47.8)	23.29 ± 3.82		26.57 ± 3.09	
More than 5000	1858 (11.6)	23.25 ± 3.89		26.78 ± 2.99	
Occupation			11.56***		8.64***
Employees	10,098 (63.1)	23.26 ± 3.81		26.52 ± 3.06	
Employers	1083 (6.8)	23.59 ± 3.90		26.93 ± 3.01	
Self-employed workers	3354 (21.0)	23.19 ± 3.95		26.70 ± 2.99	
No stable job or others	1462 (9.1)	22.73 ± 4.01		26.45 ± 3.33	
Willingness of long-term residence			5.50***		8.58***
Willing	9456 (59.1)	23.36 ± 3.88		26.75 ± 3.02	
Unwilling	6541 (40.9)	23.02 ± 3.85		26.33 ± 3.14	
Willingness of *hukou* moving			5.949***		2.55*
Willing	7935 (49.6)	23.40 ± 3.83		26.64 ± 3.10	
Unwilling	8062 (50.4)	23.043.90		26.52 ± 3.05	
Urban identity			9.56***		9.96***
Identified	14,505 (90.7)	23.31 ± 3.86		26.67 ± 3.00	
Not identified	1492 (9.3)	22.31 ± 3.83		25.70 ± 3.61	
Local acceptance			10.45***		10.41***
Accepted	14,505 (90.7)	23.32 ± 3.84		26.67 ± 2.99	

(continued)

Table 2 (continued)

Variables	n (%)	General health score		Mental health score	
		M ± SD	t/F	M ± SD	t/F
Not accepted	1492 (9.3)	22.19 ± 4.01		25.65 ± 3.69	
	Range	M ± SD	r	M ± SD	r
Age (year)	[15, 59]	32.08 ± 8.72	−0.109***	32.08 ± 8.72	0.052***
$Age^2/100$	[2.25, 34.81]	11.06 ± 6.00	−0.109***	11.06 ± 6.00	0.052***
Duration of migration (year)	[0, 41]	4.25 ± 4.43	−0.019*	4.25 ± 4.43	0.053***

Note *$p < 0.05$, **$p < 0.01$, ***$p < 0.001$. M: mean, SD: standard deviation, CNY: Chinese Yuan

to their host areas (90.7%) and the natives were willing to accept them (90.7%), and most of them were also willing to live in their host areas for a long time, (59.1%), but only half of the internal migrants were willing to move their *hukou* into their host areas (49.6%). The average general health score of the respondents was 23.22 and the average mental health score of them was 26.58, which shows a moderate-level of health of Chinese internal migrants. Details can be seen in Table 2.

Generally speaking, Chinese internal migrants who were male, younger, han nationality, unmarried, and with a rural *hukou*, a smaller range and duration of migration, a higher SES and a higher level of identity had a higher level of general health. By contrast, Chinese internal migrants who were older, married, and with a rural *hukou*, a larger duration of migration, a higher SES and a higher level of identity had a higher level of mental health. Details can be seen in Table 2.

3.2 Results of LCA

Table 3 shows that the BIC of Model 3 was the smallest, so three classes were yielded and used in this study.

Table 4 displays the conditional probabilities of four different identity variables in three latent classes. Class 1 showed a higher conditional probability in terms of the

Table 3 Results of model fitting in LCA

Models	G^2	Class.Err.	Npar	df	p	AIC	BIC
Mode 1: 1 class	1751.65	0.00	4	11	<0.001	63664.34	63695.06
Mode 2: 2 classes	576.12	0.22	9	6	<0.001	62498.81	62567.93
Mode 3: 3 classes	17.48	0.15	14	1	<0.001	61950.17	62057.69
Mode 4: 4 classes	1.95	0.24	19	−4	–	61944.64	62090.56

Note df: degree of freedom; AIC: Akaike Information Criterion; BIC: Bayesian Information Criterion

Table 4 Conditional and latent class probability of identity patterns

Identity indicators	Measuring	Conditional probability		
		Class 1 (adjective-type)	Class 2 (ambivalent-type)	Class 3 (rejected-type)
Willingness of long-term residence	Willing	0.7518	0.5078	0.3946
Willingness of *hukou* moving	Willing	0.9441	0.1019	0.3357
Local acceptance	Accepted	0.9607	0.9990	0.5528
Urban identity	Identified	0.9721	0.9718	0.5901
Latent class probability	–	0.4206	0.4086	0.1708

willingness of long-term residence and *hukou* moving, urban identity and local acceptance, so it was named as adjective-type identity. The conditional probability of Class 2 on local acceptance and urban identity was high, but the conditional probability of it on the willingness of long-term residence and *hukou* moving was relatively low. Therefore, Class 2 was named as ambivalent-type identity. Class 3 showed a slightly higher probability in terms of local acceptance and urban identity, but a lower probability in terms of the willingness of long-term residence and *hukou* moving. Thus, Class 3 was named as rejected-type identity. The latent class probability of "adjective-type identity", "ambivalent-type identity" and "rejected-type identity" was 42.06%, 40.86% and 17.08%, respectively. It is noted that both rejected- and ambivalent-type identities should belong to immature identity, indicating an imperfect status of social cohesion.

3.3 **Hukou** *Disparities in Identity Pattern*

Compared with urban-to-urban migrants, rural-to-urban migrants were more likely to involve in the transfer of multiple identity attributes in the process of migration, so the impact of identity on health may be also different between these two groups. Table 5 shows the distribution of identity patterns based on *hukou*, and it was obvious that rural-to-urban migrants, compared with urban-to-urban migrants, had a higher probability of owning ambivalent- and rejected-type identities, suggesting a lower level of identity.

Table 5 Distribution of identity patterns with different *hukou*

	Total, n (%)	Agricultural *hukou*, n (%)	Non-agricultural *hukou*, n (%)
Adjective-type	7376 (46.11)	5899 (42.88)	1477 (65.94)
Ambivalent-type	6643 (41.53)	6082 (44.21)	561 (25.04)
Rejected-type	1978 (12.36)	1776 (12.91)	202 (9.02)
Total	15,997 (100.00)	13,757 (100.00)	2240 (100.00)

Note Chi-square test value of *hukou* and identity patterns = 416.105, $p < 0.001$

3.4 Results of OLS

Table 6 shows that, without other variables controlled for in Models 1 and 2, the general health score of the respondents who belonged to ambivalent- and rejected-type identities was 0.256 point ($p < 0.001$) and 1.210 points ($p < 0.001$) lower than those who belonged to adjective-type, respectively; however, only the mental health score of the respondents who belonged to rejected-type identity was 1.029 points ($p < 0.001$) lower than those who belonged to adjective-type. By contrast, with other variables controlled for in Models 3 and 4, the general health score of the respondents who belonged to ambivalent- and rejected-type identities was 0.336 point ($p < 0.001$) and 1.312 points ($p < 0.001$) lower than those who belonged to adjective-type, respectively; and still the mental health score of the respondents who belonged to rejected-type identity was 1.024 points ($p < 0.001$) lower than those who belonged to adjective-type. Thus, the overall health performance of the internal migrants who belonged to ambivalent- and rejected-type identities was even worse compared with the respondents who belonged to adjective-type identity. The changes from Model 1 to Model 3 suggests that the impact of identity patterns on the general health of Chinese internal migrants were partly due to those differences in demographic, migration and SES factors.

A comparison between rural-to-urban and urban-to-urban migrants is displayed in Models 5 to 8. With other variables controlled for in Model 5, the general health score of the rural-to-urban migrants who belonged to ambivalent- and rejected-type identities was 0.377 point ($p < 0.001$) and 1.377 points ($p < 0.001$) lower than those who belonged to adjective-type, respectively. However, with other variables controlled for in Model 7, only the general health score of the urban-to-urban migrants who belonged to rejected-type identity was 1.168 points ($p < 0.001$) lower than those who belonged to adjective-type, and the general health score difference between ambivalent- and adjective-type identities was not statistically significant. By contrast, the mental health score of the internal migrants who belonged to rejected-type identity was 0.983 point ($p < 0.001$) and 1.309 points ($p < 0.001$) lower than those who belonged to adjective-type in rural-to-urban and urban-to-urban migrants, respectively. Thus, adjective-type identity was a protective factor for health in Chinese internal migrants.

In addition to identity patterns, some significant associations were also observed between other variables and two health outcomes. Age was inversely associated with general health, and every additional unit of age increased general health by 0.095. Chinese internal migrants being male and with Han nationality, agricultural *hukou* and a smaller range of migration had a higher general health score. Although a higher occupational status was related to better general health, more education was strangely related to poorer general health. For mental health, it is observed that there was a U-shaped association between age and mental health; Chinese internal migrants being married, with a larger duration of migration, more personal income and a higher occupational status had better mental health.

4 Discussion

The health of Chinese internal migrants has always been paid much attention to, and scholars have gradually focused on social cohesion for health in recent years. Many studies have found that social cohesion has a protective effect on migrants' health (Fothergill et al., 2011; Wang & Chen, 2015). In the process of social integration to the new life in cities, migrants gain environmental adaptability and identity on the basis of enough material conditions, which is further conducive to the acquisition of material and spiritual resources (Cohen, 2004) and the improvement of their health. Therefore, social cohesion is considered an important social determinant of health (Zhang, Chen, & Ma, 2015). As an important component of social cohesion, identity also closely relates to migrants' health.

Prior studies indicate that social cohesion has a lagging effect on migrants' health (Meng, Li, & Su, 2019), and there are also SES disparities in the association between social cohesion and health (Yang et al., 2016). It is observed that the adverse effect of SES constraints on health can be alleviated by social cohesion, and, as a key component of social cohesion, identity is positively related to the SES of migrants (Pan & He, 2017). The results of LCA show that most Chinese internal migrants belonged to adjective- and ambivalent-type identities (42.1% and 40.9%, respectively), which is basically in line with the results of Hou and Yao's study (Hou & Yao, 2016). With other variables controlled for, adjective-type identity was a protective factor of health for Chinese internal migrants, while ambivalent- and rejected-type identities were not significantly related to their health. Identity pattern is a valid predictor of health of Chinese internal migrants. Adjective-type identity is a strong sense of identity and belonging to urban life, which is conducive to migrants' health. By contrast, ambivalent- and rejected-type identities are immature types of identity, and migrants belonging to them are easy to experience more contradictions and confusions and unable to establish a good sense of belonging, so they may suffer from more health problems.

Previous evidence suggests that, in China, *hukou* system may weaken the social cohesion between urban locals and migrants and strengthen discrimination and bias (Shi, Dang, Zheng, & Liu, 2017). Low-level identity, institutional exclusion and

Table 6 Influencing factors of health status: based on OLS

Variables	Model 1	Model 2	Model 3	Model 4	Model 5	Model 6	Model 7	Model 8
	General health	Mental health	General health	Mental health	General health	Mental health	General health	Mental health
Identity patterns (ref: adjective-type)								
Ambivalent-type	−0.256***(0.065)	−0.051(0.053)	−0.336***(0.066)	−0.079(0.053)	−0.377***(0.070)	−0.074(0.056)	−0.031(0.197)	−0.024(0.167)
Rejected-type	−1.210***(0.097)	−1.029***(0.077)	−1.312***(0.098)	−1.024***(0.078)	−1.337***(0.104)	−0.983***(0.082)	−1.168***(0.294)	−1.309***(0.248)
Hukou (ref: non-agricultural)			0.219*(0.097)	0.146(0.077)				
Ethnicity (ref: Han nationality)			−0.325*(0.165)	0.210(0.132)	−0.302(0.177)	0.195(0.140)	−0.533(0.463)	0.161(0.392)
Gender (ref: male)			−0.471***(0.064)	−0.020(0.051)	−0.496***(0.069)	−0.050(0.055)	−0.275(0.172)	0.164(0.145)
Marital status (ref: married)			−0.027(0.095)	−0.446***(0.076)	0.047(0.105)	−0.412***(0.083)	−0.394(0.231)	−0.546**(0.196)
Age			−0.095**(0.028)	−0.074**(0.022)	−0.087**(0.030)	−0.065**(0.024)	−0.070(0.078)	−0.092(0.066)
$Age^2/100$			0.053(0.039)	0.106**(0.031)	0.042(0.042)	0.088**(0.033)	0.026(0.106)	0.159(0.089)
Duration of migration			0.011(0.007)	0.022***(0.006)	0.008(0.008)	0.029***(0.006)	0.024(0.019)	−0.013(0.016)
Range of migration (ref: inter-provincial)								
Cross-city within province			0.076(0.064)	0.091(0.051)	0.064(0.069)	0.141**(0.054)	0.102(0.183)	−0.156(0.155)
Cross-county within city			0.515**(0.163)	0.252(0.130)	0.463*(0.182)	0.220(0.144)	0.664(0.374)	0.428(0.316)
Education (ref: primary school or below)								
Junior high school			0.048(0.113)	0.092(0.090)	0.053(0.116)	0.030(0.092)	−0.488(0.497)	0.824*(0.420)
Senior high school			−0.108(0.125)	−0.182(0.090)	−0.089(0.131)	−0.252*(0.104)	−0.804(0.494)	0.690(0.417)
College or above			−0.621***(0.145)	−0.212(0.116)	−0.595***(0.160)	−0.423**(0.127)	−1.094*(0.498)	0.893*(0.421)
Personal income monthly (ref: less than 3000)								
3000 to 5000			0.046(0.071)	0.028(0.057)	0.094(0.076)	0.041(0.060)	−0.357(0.220)	−0.047(0.186)
More than 5000			0.021(0.113)	0.215*(0.091)	0.112(0.127)	0.132(0.101)	−0.453(0.277)	0.376(0.234)

(continued)

Table 6 (continued)

Variables	Model 1	Model 2	Model 3	Model 4	Model 5	Model 6	Model 7	Model 8
	General health	Mental health	General health	Mental health	General health	Mental health	General health	Mental health
Occupation (ref: no stable job or others)								
Employees			0.360**(0.115)	0.164(0.092)	0.333**(0.124)	0.191*(0.098)	0.664*(0.314)	0.026(0.265)
Employers			0.806***(0.163)	0.341**(0.130)	0.657***(0.177)	0.310*(0.140)	1.689***(0.426)	0.632(0.360)
Self-employed workers			0.348**(0.129)	0.105(0.103)	0.326*(0.138)	0.126(0.109)	0.555(0.371)	0.077(0.313)
Adjusted R^2	0.009	0.012	0.033	0.020	0.034	0.020	0.021	0.027
n	15,997		15,997		13,757		2240	

Note Standard error in parentheses; $*p < 0.05$, $**p < 0.01$, $***p < 0.001$

cultural barriers caused by *hukou* are core factors that lead to the dilemma of social cohesion for rural-to-urban migrants (Cui, 2012). Thus, urban-to-urban migrants may be more agreeable to their city identity (Li & Zhang, 2019), which is more conducive to their health. By contrast, rural-to-urban migrants are more likely to fall into the dilemma of identity, and some of them may have a contradictory understanding on urban identity, which is not conducive to their health. The results of this study also show that ambivalent-type identity was only related to the general health of rural-to-urban migrants, but rejected-type identity was related to the general and mental health of both rural-to-urban and urban-to-urban migrants. This suggests that the identity transition and group role attribution formed by rural-to-urban migrants after they migrate to cities have a positive impact on their health. The *hukou* system indeed hinders the social cohesion of Chinese internal migrants. Therefore, rural-to-urban migrants with ambivalent- and rejected-type identities are more likely to have a poorer general health status, while only urban-to-urban migrants with rejected-type identity suffer from more health problems.

The aforementioned results provide some suggestive things, and some intervention strategies are proposed accordingly. First, because most Chinese internal migrants are rural-to-urban migrants, local residents in urban areas need to respect them and reduce their discrimination against migrants. Local governments need to strengthen community constructions and functions and make the community a platform for communication between rural-to-urban migrants and the natives in urban areas. Policymakers should also formulate and carry out relevant policies for this unique group, such as boosting the reform of the household registration system and equally providing basic living conditions and healthcare services/resources for rural-to-urban migrants, to help them integrate into urban lives more easily. On the other hand, Chinese internal migrants themselves should strengthen the sense of belonging and identity, they should actively participate in community activities in their host areas. Furthermore, internal migrants should also strive to improve their working skills and seek institutional guarantees, thus laying the foundation for better social cohesion.

Several limitations can be found in this study. First, this is a cross-sectional study, and OLS is used, so the association between identity and health may not be causal. Second, although this study uses LCA to analyze the correlation between different identity variables, there are still many other behavioral variables that may involve the connotation of identity. Only four variables are extracted, and a more comprehensive study is needed in the future.

5 Conclusion

Most Chinese internal migrants belong to adjective- and ambivalent-type identities. Rural-to-urban migrants are more likely to have ambivalent-type identity, while, urban-to-urban migrants are more likely to have adjective-type identity. Adjective-type identity is an important protective factor for the health of both urban-to-urban and rural-to-urban migrants, but ambivalent-type identity only adversely relates to general health in rural-to-urban migrants. Some interventions should be conducted to improve the social cohesion of internal migrants in China to promote their health.

References

Bracke, P. F. (2001). Measuring the subjective well-being of people in a psychosocial rehabilitation center and a residential psychiatric setting: The outline of the study and the measurement properties of a multidimensional indicator of well-being. *Psychiatric Rehabilitation Journal, 24*(3), 222–236.

Chen, Y., Zhang, L., & Yu, X. (2018). Study on the relationship between migrant workers' children in the city's self-evaluation, social identity and mental health. *Journal of Qiqihar University (Philosophy and Social Sciences Edition)* (2), 57–59.

Cohen, S. (2004). Social relationships and health. *American Psychologist, 59*(8), 676–684.

Cui, Y. (2012). A study on migrants' psychological integration and self-identity. *Sociological Studies* (5), 141–160.

Fothergill, K. E., Ensminger, M. E., Robertson, J., Green, K. M., Thorpe, R. J., & Juon, H.-S. (2011). Effects of social integration on health: A prospective study of community engagement among African American women. *Social Science and Medicine, 72*(2), 291–298.

Fromm, E. (2001). *The sane society*. London: Routledge.

Guo, X., & Xing, Z. (2009). The inherent two-dimensional diagram of social identification: A case study of social identification of off-farm workers in Beijing. *Jiangsu Social Sciences* (4), 54–60.

Hale, C. J., Hannum, J. W., & Espelage, D. L. (2005). Social support and physical health: The importance of belonging. *Journal of American College Health, 53*(6), 276–284.

Hou, Y., & Yao, H. (2016). Patterns of migrant identity: A latent class analysis. *Population Research, 40*(2), 38–49.

Jiang, J., & Wang, P. (2018). Health status in a transitional society: Urban-rural disparities from a dynamic perspective in China. *Population Health Metrics, 16*, e22.

Lairson, D. R., Hindson, P., & Hauquitz, A. (1995). Equity of health care in Australia. *Social Science and Medicine, 41*(4), 475–482.

Li, B., & Zhang, G. (2019). Logic of identity differentiation for the agricultural transfer population. *Sociological Studies* (3), 146–169.

Li, R., & Zhang, L. (2012). A study of floating population self-identity present situation and its influence factor: Based on the survey data of 106 cities in our country. *Population and Economics* (4), 78–86.

Lin, T. H., & Dayton, C. M. (1997). Model selection information criteria for non-nested latent class models. *Journal of Education and Behavioral Statistics, 22*(3), 249–264.

Meng, F., Li, T., & Su, Z. (2019). A study on the influence of urban integration on the physical health of rural migrant workers. *Journal of Ocean University of China (Social Sciences)* (4), 104–113.

National Bureau of Statistics. (2018). *China statistical yearbook 2017*. Beijing: China Statistics Press.

Pan, Z., & He, Q. (2017). Living space, social communication and subjective status cognition: Research on the identity of migrant workers. *Social Sciences in Hunan* (1), 80–87.

Qiu, Z. (2008). *Latent class model: Principles and techniques*. Beijing: Educational Science Publishing House.

Shan, D. (2011). *Social identity of urban migrant children and its impact on mental health*. Xian: Shaanxi Normal University.

Shi, Y. (2016). Household registration system and family reunion. *Youth Studies* (6), 11–20.

Shi, Y., Dang, J., Zheng, W., & Liu, L. (2017). Dual identity and prejudice: The moderating role of group boundary permeability. *Frontiers in Psychology, 8*, e195.

Tajfel, H. E. (1978). *Differentiation between social groups: Studies in the social psychology of inter-group relations*. London: Academic Press.

Tang, J., & Li, J. (2019). The concepts of overall health and health management from a health sociology perspective. *Social Sciences in China* (8), 130–148.

Wang, P. (2016). *Report on China's migrant population development*. Beijing: China Population Publishing House.

Wang, P., & Chen, X. (2015). Social capital, social cohesion and health attainment: taking example for rural-to-urban migrants. *Journal of Huazhong University of Science and Technology (Social Science Edition), 29*(3), 81–88.

Wang, S., Fan, W., Yu, W., Li, J., Xu, D., Cao, H., et al. (2016). Analysis of reliability and validity of SF-36 scale in urban residents. *Chinese Journal of Epidemiology, 37*(3), 344–347.

Ware, J. E., & Gandek, B. (1998). Overview of the SF-36 health survey and the international quality of life assessment (IQOLA) project. *Journal of Clinical Epidemiology, 51*(11), 903–912.

Xu, H., Xiong, H., Chen, Y., Wang, L., Liu, T., et al. (2013). The application of the Chinese version of K6 and K10 screening scales for psychological distress on the psychological investigation of college students. *Modern Preventive Medicine, 40*(24), 4493–4496.

Yan, Z., Peng, A., Liu, F., & Zhang, L. (2009). Analysis on the relationship of social support, body health and perceived health of floating population from rural area. *Modern Preventive Medicine, 36*(5), 892–894 + 899.

Yang, J., Zhang, J., & Zhang, Z. (2016). Interactive mechanism of the floating population's health equity and social integration. *Chinese Journal of Health Policy, 9*(8), 66–74.

Yu, H., & Yu, L. (2018). Social convergence, social support and health of floating population: An empirical analysis based on Zhejiang. *Zhejiang Social Sciences* (6), 86–95.

Zhang, C., Chen, J., & Ma, X. (2015). Social integration and health promotion in floating population. *Modern Preventive Medicine, 42*(8), 1519–1522.

Zheng, W., Xu, L., Zhou, C., & Li, X. (2009). Application of Kessler 10 rating scale in study on relationship between accidental injury and mental health status. *Chinese Mental Health Journal* (3), 175–178.

Chapter 6
Economic Factors and Life Satisfaction in Internal Migrants: A Moderated Mediation Model of Perceived Stress and Social Integration

Peigang Wang, Yayun Xu, and Ling Zhang

1 Introduction

In China, internal migrants accounts for a considerable proportion of the national population. With the development of industrialization and urbanization in China, the scale of internal migrants keeps increasing. Improving the living condition and happiness of internal migrants has been one of the major missions of China's population policy. Therefore, researching on how to improve the life satisfaction of internal migrants is immensely important in China.

Life satisfaction is the subjective evaluation reflecting the feelings one has about the quality of his or her life. In a meta-analytic attempt to define the multiple domains of life satisfaction, Cummins (1996) categorized satisfaction into seven broad domains, including emotional well-being, health, intimacy, material well-being, safety, community, and productivity. Life satisfaction or happiness is commonly known as a main goal for human beings (Eid & Larsen, 2008; Sanders & Maria, 2014) and identifying the factors associated with it can therefore be considered important as well (Herbers & Mulder, 2017).

Previous studies have confirmed that economic factors are important factors affecting people's life satisfaction. According to previous studies, housing satisfaction has a strongly positive impact on life satisfaction, and housing satisfaction as well as homeownership is an important factor determining overall happiness. More concretely, permanent housing and better amenities may contribute to housing satisfaction and life satisfaction (Tuyen & Vu, 2018; Zhang, Zhang, & Hudson, 2018). Prior studies

P. Wang (✉) · L. Zhang
Population and Health Research Center, School of Health Sciences,
Wuhan University, Wuhan, China
e-mail: wpg926@whu.edu.cn

Y. Xu
Hangzhou Tigermed Consulting Co., Ltd, Hangzhou, China

P. Wang (ed.), *The Health Status of Internal Migrants in China*,
https://doi.org/10.1007/978-981-15-4415-6_6

indicate that income is an important factor that contributes to a higher level of life satisfaction (Howell & Howell, 2008; Kahneman & Deaton, 2010; Lucas & Dyrenforth, 2006). Gere and Schimmack (2017) verified money-increases-happiness hypothesis. Ambrey and Fleming (2014) further confirmed the causal effect of income on life satisfaction. There is also an analysis revealing the association between higher pessimism/stress levels and lower life satisfaction in people who are unemployed (Haid & Seiffge-Krenke, 2013). Findings of Hessels (2018) reveal that self-employed workers are more satisfied with their lives than paid employees, and self-employment can help to reduce the situation of low life satisfaction associated with blue-collar and low-skilled work.

The influential factors of life satisfaction have been widely discussed. However, the pathway through which these factors affect life satisfaction is less-frequently researched. Since these factors can act as potential stressors, in this chapter, we introduced perceived stress as the mediator between economic factors and life satisfaction.

Stress has long been a major research concept in health science, as it links to various adverse psychological, biological, and behavioral outcomes (Joseph & Golden, 2017; Turpin et al., 2019; Wiegner et al., 2015). Life satisfaction is a judgmental process in which individuals assess the quality of their lives based on a variety of criteria (Pavot & Diener, 2009). Thus, life satisfaction can be influenced by the combination of stress and its adverse outcomes. Prior studies have found that perceived stress has a negative impact on life satisfaction (Alleyne, Alleyne, & Greenidge, 2010; Extremera, Duran, & Rey, 2009; Rupert & Hawi, 2016). Shi (2015) also found that more perceived stress would cause lower levels of life satisfaction through lower levels of resilience.

Many studies have found a correlation between economic factors and perceived stress (Alleyne et al., 2010; Eskin et al., 2014; Extremera et al., 2009; J. Li & Z. Liu, 2018; Rey & Extremera, 2015; Rossi & Bisconti, 2003; Sehlen et al., 2009; Yoo, 2016). The coping theory suggests that stress arises when an individual perceives that he or she does not have adequate resources to cope with current or anticipatory demands (Lazarus & Folkman, 1984). Previous study (J. Li & Z. Liu, 2018) also find that poor housing conditions are significantly associated with more perceived stress. As they point out, informal housing tenants lead to the highest level of perceived stress and worst mental health compared to dormitory tenants and formal housing residents. Based on these findings, we propose the following hypotheses.

Hypothesis 1: Economic factors can affect the level of life satisfaction in internal migrants.

Hypothesis 2: Perceived stress plays a mediating role in the process of economic factors affecting life satisfaction.

Although economic factors are generally related to life satisfaction, the life satisfaction of internal migrants may not be equally influenced by economic factors. Consequently, it is important to examine factors that may moderate the relationship between economic factors and life satisfaction. Moving into a new environment, the internal migrants have to decide how to interact with the natives around them and this decision greatly determines their social integration. Social integration indicates the quality of social relationships established and social supports people can receive (Turner & Turner, 2013). The study of Nabi (2013) shows that even online relationships (number of Facebook friends) can reduce stress and have health benefit. These can provide adequate resources to cope with the individuals' current or anticipatory demands. For example, Schwarzer (2014) found that social integration buffers the impact of stressors on stress responses. Based on previous studies, we propose the following hypothesis.

Hypothesis 3: The mediating effect of perceived stress between economic factors and life satisfaction is moderated by social integration.

2 Data and Methods

2.1 Participants

The data used in the present study are from a sub-study of the China Migrants Dynamic Survey (CMDS) in 2014. The topic of the sub-study was the social integration and mental health of internal migrants. Eight cities were selected to conduct the sub-study from the sample cities of CMDS and the participants were sampled within these cities by a PPS (Probability Proportionate to Size Sampling) method. The participants were internal migrants who had been living in the sample area for at least one month and were 15–59 years of age. With missing data deleted using a list-wise method, the data used for analysis in the present study came from 15,997 participants.

2.2 Measurements

Life satisfaction was measured using the Chinese edition of the Satisfaction With Life Scale (SWLS) (Pavot & Diener, 1993, 2009; Wang, Yuen, & Slaney, 2008). The SWLS is a short 5-item instrument designed to measure cognitive judgments of satisfaction with one's life. An example of an item from the SWLS is "In most ways my life is close to my ideal." Participants were asked to rate items on a 7-point Likert-type scale ranging from 1 (strongly disagree) to 7 (strongly agree). Higher scores indicate higher life satisfaction. The Cronbach's alpha for the SWLS is 0.86. The sum scores of five items were calculated (ranging from 5 to 35) to reflect participants' life satisfaction.

Perceived stress was assessed by the Perceived Stress Scale-4 (PSS-4) (Cohen, Kamarck, & Mermelstein, 1983). The PSS-4 consists of 4 items asking the participants about their feelings and thoughts over the past month. Each item is rated from 0 (never) to 4 (very often). The Scores of two items, "how often have you felt confident about your ability to handle your personal problems" and "how often have you felt that things are going your way", are inversed for the purpose that a higher score reflect a higher level of perceived stress. The Cronbach's alpha for the SWLS is 0.60. The Sum scores of four items were calculated (ranging from 0 to 16) to reflect participants' perceived stress.

Social integration was assessed using the Social Integration Scale of Internal Migrants, which was developed for the CMDS in 2014 and was validated by Tang (Tang, 2015). This 4-item scale reflects the level of social integration by rating from 1 (strongly disagree) to 4 (strongly agree). An example of an item is "I feel belongingness to the city where I live now". The Cronbach's alpha for the Social Integration Scale of Internal Migrants was 0.67 in Tang's study (Tang, 2015) and 0.68 in the present study. The sum scores of four items were calculated (ranging from 4 to 16) and a higher score means a higher level of social integration.

Predicting variables are economic status which include housing type ("Rented", "Owned", "Provided without paying" and "Other"), employment ("Employee", "Employer", "Self-employed", "None" and "Others"), personal monthly income (Chinese Yuan, CNY) ("0", "≤3000", "≤4500", ">4500").

2.3 *Statistical Analysis*

Descriptive statistics were used to summarize the characteristics of participants and main variables in the present study. The mediation models and moderated mediation models were tested by the SAS macro "PROCESS" (version 3.0) developed by Hayes, which can deal with models with multi-categorical predictor variables (Hayes, 2018). Figure 1a presents the conceptual diagram of the mediation model. In the present study, the predictor variable is economic factors, the mediator variable is perceived stress, and the outcome variable is life satisfaction.

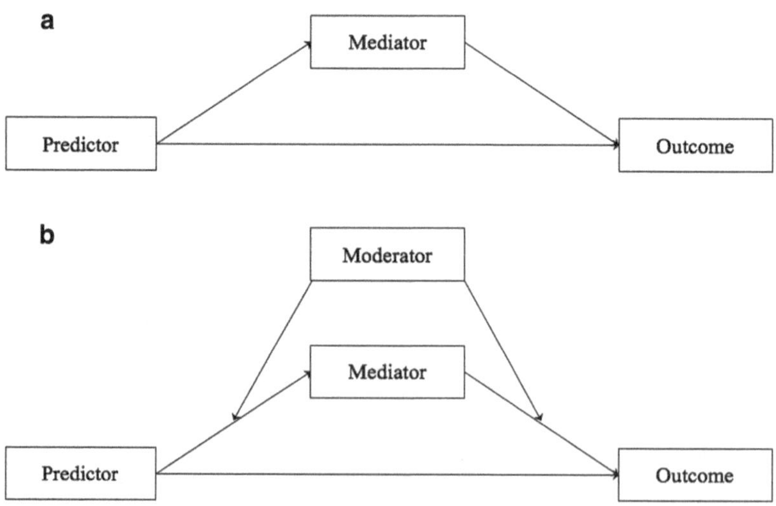

Fig. 1 Conceptual diagram for mediation model (**a**) and moderated mediation model (**b**)

As shown in Fig. 1a, the direct effects of the predictor variable (economic factors in this study) on the outcome variable (life satisfaction in this study), the predictor variable on the mediator variable (perceived stress in this study), and the mediator variable on the outcome variable will be estimated. Meanwhile, the indirect effect of the predictor variable on the outcome variable through the mediator variable will also be estimated. The 95% confidence interval is provided by the bootstrapping method. Figure 1b presents the conceptual diagram of the moderated mediation model that is tested in the present study. In this model, the effects of the predictor variable on the mediator variable, and the mediator variable on the outcome variable are moderated by a common moderator variable, that is, social integration in the present study. The indirect effect of the predictor variable on the outcome variable through the mediator variable is conditional on different level of the moderator variable. For example, the indirect effect of the predictor variable on the outcome variable through the mediator variable is stronger at a higher level of the moderator variable than that at a lower level of the moderator variable. This SAS macro has been widely used in prior studies (Gray et al., 2015; Zhou et al., 2017).

All analyses were completed using SAS version 9.4 (SAS Institute, Cary, NC).

3 Results

3.1 Sample Characteristics

The data used for final analysis came from 15,997 participants (8798 males and 7199 females), with a mean age of 32.7 (standard deviation (SD) = 8.7, ranging from 15 to 59 years). 54.8% of the participants (8769) were moving across provinces, and 41.4% of them (6625) were moving within a province, only 3.8% of them (593) were moving within a city. A majority of them (12,135, 75.9%) had an education of junior or senior high school, and 14.7% of them (2358) had an education of college or above. There were still 9.4% participants (1504) with an education of primary school or below. The median of the duration of migration was 7 years, ranging from 0 (less than 1 year) to 44 years. 86.0% (13,757) of the participants hold an agricultural *hukou* (household registration system of China) and the others hold a non-agricultural *hukou*.

3.2 Preliminary Analysis

The mean scores of life satisfaction, perceived stress and social integration were 21.8 ($SD = 6.25$), 9.3 ($SD = 2.64$) and 12.8 ($SD = 1.95$), respectively. Life satisfaction was negatively related to perceived stress ($r = -0.379$, $p < 0.001$) and positively

Table 1 Relationship between perceived stress, life satisfaction and social integration

	Mean	SD	1	2	3
1. Life satisfaction	21.8	6.25	–		
2. Perceived stress	9.3	2.64	−0.379***	–	
3. Social integration	12.8	1.95	0.176***	−0.227***	–

Note Values in the table are Pearson correlation coefficients. $^{*}p < 0.05$, $^{**}p < 0.01$, $^{***}p < 0.001$

related to social integration ($r = 0.176$, $p < 0.001$). Perceived stress was negatively related to social integration ($r = -0.227$, $p < 0.001$) (Table 1).

Table 2 presents the relationships between economic status, covariates and both of perceived stress and life satisfaction. The migrants who had owned or bought a house or an apartment, or who was an employer, or who had the highest income, or who participated in different types of social activities had the lowest perceived stress and the highest life satisfaction. Older migrants tended to have lower perceived stress and higher life satisfaction than younger ones. Male migrants had lower perceived stress and lower life satisfaction than female ones. Migrants with less education or with non-agricultural *hukou* had better life satisfaction. The larger the range of migration (not geographical distance, across provinces > within a province > within a city) was, the higher the perceived stress was. Migrants who were not married had the highest perceived stress and lowest life satisfaction. Migrants with a longer duration of migration tended to have lower perceived stress and higher life satisfaction.

3.3 Moderated Mediation Model

Table 3 shows that, compared with migrants who rented a place to live in, those who owned a house or an apartment had lower perceived stress ($\beta = -0.46$, $p < 0.001$), which could then cause higher life satisfaction ($\beta = -0.87$, $p < 0.001$). The relative mediation effect of owning a house on life satisfaction through decreased perceived stress was 0.40 (95%CI: 0.28, 0.52). Compared with employees, employers had lower perceived stress ($\beta = -0.50$, $p < 0.001$), which could then cause higher life satisfaction ($\beta = -0.87$, $p < 0.001$). The relative mediation effect of being employers on life satisfaction through decreased perceived stress was 0.44 (95%CI: 0.29, 0.60). Self-employment also improved life satisfaction mediated by decreased perceived stress, and the relative mediation effect was 0.14 (95%CI: 0.05, 0.24). Compared with lower personal income ($\leq$3000 CNY), the relative mediation effect of personal income between 3000 to 4500 CNY on life satisfaction through decreased perceived stress was 0.24 (95%CI: 0.15, 0.34), and the relative mediation effect of personal income higher than 4500 CNY on life satisfaction through decreased perceived stress was 0.45 (95%CI: 0.34, 0.55). Among all the X variables, only the effect of personal income between 3000 to 4500 CNY (relative to $\leq$3000 CNY) was fully mediated by perceived stress, as the direct effect was 0.18 ($p > 0.05$). For the other variables, the

Table 2 Relationship between economic status, covariates and perceived stress, life satisfaction

Migration related factors	n	Perceived stress	Life satisfaction
		Mean (SD)	Mean (SD)
Economic			
Housing type			
Rented	12,424	9.4 (2.63)***	21.6 (6.19)***
Owned	1584	8.7 (2.65)	24.4 (6.00)
Provided without paying	1663	9.4 (2.60)	21.2 (6.25)
Other	326	9.2 (2.66)	21.2 (6.83)
Employment			
Employee	10,098	9.4 (2.60)***	21.3 (6.14)***
Employer	1083	8.8 (2.71)	23.8 (6.19)
Self-employed	3354	9.1 (2.67)	22.6 (6.24)
None	1330	9.4 (2.67)	22.3 (6.48)
Other	132	9.3 (2.76)	22.0 (7.84)
Income (CNY)			
No income	1225	9.3 (2.70)***	22.4 (6.48)***
≤3000	7963	9.5 (2.60)	21.3 (6.22)
≤4500	3689	9.2 (2.60)	21.7 (6.02)
>4500	3120	8.9 (2.70)	23.1 (6.32)
Covariates			
Age			
≤25	3660	9.5 (2.59)***	20.8 (6.19)***
≤35	6687	9.3 (2.62)	21.8 (6.20)
≤45	4211	9.2 (2.68)	22.5 (6.30)
≤55	1304	9.0 (2.65)	22.9 (6.05)
>55	135	9.0 (2.94)	22.6 (6.37)
Gender			
Male	8798	9.2 (2.64)*	21.7 (6.28)**
Female	7199	9.3 (2.64)	22.0 (6.21)
Education			
Primary school or below	1504	9.3 (2.67)	22.4 (6.24)***
Junior or senior high school	12,135	9.3 (2.63)	21.8 (6.25)
University/Collage or above	2358	9.2 (2.63)	21.7 (6.21)
Hukou			
Agricultural	13,757	9.3 (2.63)	21.8 (6.23)***
Non-agricultural	2240	9.2 (2.68)	22.3 (6.34)
Range of migration			

(continued)

Table 2 (continued)

Migration related factors	n	Perceived stress	Life satisfaction
		Mean (SD)	Mean (SD)
Across provinces	8769	9.4 (2.63)***	21.8 (6.22)
Within a province	6635	9.2 (2.64)	21.8 (6.28)
Within a city	593	8.9 (2.64)	22.3 (6.27)
Number of children			
0	793	9.3 (2.69)***	21.9 (6.16)***
1	6464	9.2 (2.63)	22.4 (61.7)
≥2	4684	9.2 (2.67)	22.3 (6.26)
Not married	4056	9.6 (2.58)	20.4 (6.16)
Duration of migration (Years)			
≤5	6375	9.5 (2.62)***	21.4 (6.23)***
≤10	4232	9.3 (2.62)	21.7 (6.21)
>10	5390	9.1 (2.65)	22.4 (6.25)

Note All analyses were performed using ANOVA. *$p < 0.05$, **$p < 0.01$, ***$p < 0.001$. SD: standard deviation

direct effects were all stronger than mediation effects. For example, the direct effect of owning a house on life satisfaction was 1.96 ($p < 0.001$) and it was stronger than mediation effect through perceived stress which was 0.40 (95%CI: 0.28, 0.52).

Figure 2 presents the moderated mediation models in Table 3. The coefficients in Fig. 2 are corresponding to the effects shown in Fig. 1b. For example, in Fig. 2a, the main effect between housing and perceived stress was no longer significant while the moderation effect was. With one score increase of social integration, the effect (absolute effect size) of owning a house on perceived stress would increase by 0.08. This indicates that among those with higher social integration, the relationship between housing and perceived stress will be stronger. Similarly, the effect (absolute effect size) of perceived stress on life satisfaction would increase by 0.02 with one score increase of social integration. This two moderation effects would result in increased indirect effect of owning a house on life satisfaction through perceived stress.

The moderation effect of social integration on the relationship between perceived stress and life satisfaction was significant with $p < 0.01$. This moderation effect exists in all mediation models tested in this study. For type of housing, the effect of owing a house or an apartment on perceived stress was also moderated by social integration. The SAS macro PROCESS provided indirect effect at different levels of the moderator. At a higher level of social integration, the indirect effect of owing a house or an apartment on life satisfaction through perceived stress was 0.36 (95%CI: 0.20, 0.53). But the indirect effect, 0.08 (95%CI: −0.11, 0.26), was no longer significant at a lower level of social integration. The following indirect effect were also moderated by social integration: the indirect effect of being an employer on life satisfaction through perceived stress, compared with being an employee; the indirect

Table 3 Results of mediation models and moderated mediation models

Migration related factors	Social integration	X → M	M → Y	X → Y	X → M → Y
Housing ("Rented" as ref.)					
Owned	Overall	−0.46***	−0.87***	1.96***	**0.40 (0.28, 0.52)**
	High	−0.42***+	−0.87***+	1.80***	**0.36 (0.20, 0.53)**
	Low	−0.10	−0.78***	1.80***	0.08 (−0.11, 0.26)
Provided without paying	Overall	−0.09	−0.87***+	−0.20	0.08 (−0.04, 0.20)
	High	−0.16	−0.87***	−0.21	0.14 (−0.05, 0.32)
	Low	−0.02	−0.78***	−0.21	0.02 (−0.11, 0.15)
Other	Overall	−0.11	−0.87***	−0.68*	0.10 (−0.16, 0.35)
	High	−0.34++	−0.87***+	−0.83**	0.30 (−0.02, 0.63)
	Low	0.48*	−0.78***	−0.83**	**−0.38 (−0.65, −0.08)**
Employment ("Employee" as ref.)					
Employer	Overall	−0.50***	−0.87***	1.63***	**0.44 (0.29, 0.60)**
	High	−0.53***	−0.87***++	1.52***	**0.46 (0.25, 0.67)**
	Low	−0.25*	−0.78***	1.52***	**0.19 (0.01, 0.39)**
Self-employed	Overall	−0.16**	−0.87***	0.66***	**0.14 (0.05, 0.24)**
	High	−0.20*	−0.87***++	0.63***	**0.17 (0.03, 0.32)**
	Low	−0.07	−0.78***	0.63***	0.05 (−0.05, 0.17)
None	Overall	0.01	−0.87***	0.44*	−0.01 (−0.14, 0.13)
	High	−0.10	−0.87***++	0.45**	0.09 (−0.13, 0.30)
	Low	0.05	−0.78***	0.45**	−0.04 (−0.19, 0.11)
Other	Overall	−0.04	−0.87***	0.45	0.03 (−0.37, 0.45)

(continued)

Table 3 (continued)

Migration related factors	Social integration	X → M	M → Y	X → Y	X → M → Y
	High	−0.83*+	−0.87***++	0.51	**0.73 (0.15, 1.29)**
	Low	0.25	−0.78***	0.51	−0.20 (−0.60, 0.23)
Income (CNY) ('≤3000' as ref.)					
≤4500	Overall	−0.28***	−0.87***	0.18	**0.24 (0.15, 0.34)**
	High	−0.30***	−0.87***++	0.22	**0.26 (0.12, 0.40)**
	Low	−0.30***	−0.78***	0.22	**0.23 (0.13, 0.34)**
>4500	Overall	−0.51***	−0.87***	1.22***	**0.45 (0.34, 0.55)**
	High	−0.64***++	−0.87***++	1.21***	**0.56 (0.40, 0.71)**
	Low	−0.34***	−0.78***	1.21***	**0.27 (0.15, 0.39)**
No income	Overall	−0.10	−0.87***	0.55**	0.08 (−0.06, 0.23)
	High	−0.27*	−0.87***++	0.58**	**0.23 (0.01, 0.46)**
	Low	−0.02	−0.78***	0.58**	0.02 (−0.14, 0.18)

Note X indicates each migration related factor. M indicates the mediator which is perceived stress. Y indicates the outcome variable which is life satisfaction. "X → M" indicates the effect of X on M. "M → Y" indicates the effect of M on Y. "X → Y" indicates the direct effect of X on Y. "X → M → Y" indicates the indirect effect or mediation effect of X on Y through M. All models were controlled for age, gender, education, range of migration, number of children and duration of migration. In the 2nd column, "Overall" indicates the mediation model. "High" and "Low" indicate the mediation model in the condition where social integration was at a high level (social integration score ≥15) or a low level (social integration score ≤11), respectively. * indicates the statistical significance of the corresponding coefficient. + indicates the statistical significance of the moderation of social integration in corresponding path, X on M or M on Y. *$p < 0.05$, **$p < 0.01$, ***$p < 0.001$. +$p < 0.05$, ++$p < 0.01$, +++$p < 0.001$

effect of being self-employed on life satisfaction through perceived stress, compared with being an employee; the indirect effect of income from 3000 to 4500 CNY on life satisfaction through perceived stress, compared with income no more than 3000 CNY; the indirect effect of income higher than 4500 CNY on life satisfaction through perceived stress, compared with income no more than 3000 CNY.

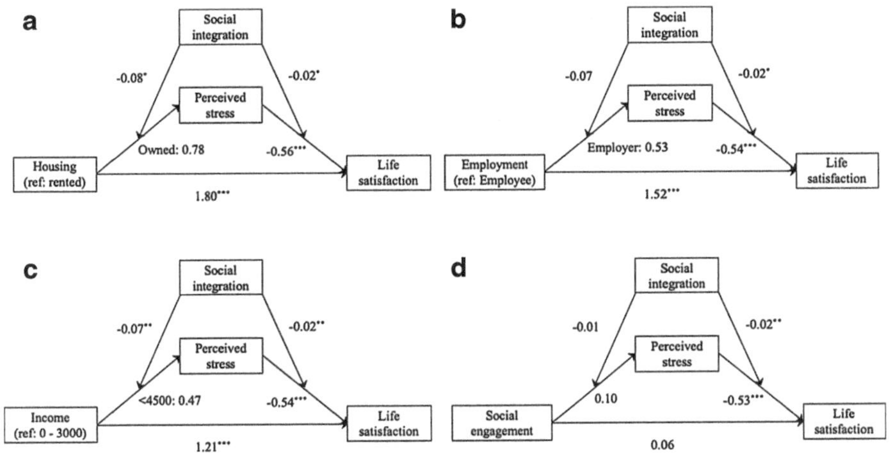

Fig. 2 Results of moderated mediation models in the present study. *Note* Only one category of predictor variables is presented in figure **a**, **b**, and **c** to show moderated mediation models. *$p < 0.05$, **$p < 0.01$, ***$p < 0.001$

4 Discussion

Life satisfaction scores are influenced both by personal factors in people's lives such as their family life and work, as well as by community and social circumstances (Diener, Inglehart, & Tay, 2013). Thus, life satisfaction can provide an additional window on what is going well or badly in a society, as experienced by the citizens themselves. The main purpose of this study is to explore how economic factors influence life satisfaction among internal migrants in China, by testing the mediation effect of perceived stress and the moderation effect of social integration. From the policy maker's perspective, the results can provide a new basis to further understand the mechanism of life satisfaction of internal migrants in China, and also provide evidence to improve the quality of life among Chinese internal migrants.

The results, consistent with Hypothesis 2, show that the economic factors can be linked to life satisfaction via perceived stress in the internal migrants in China. In previous studies, the relationships between these three aspects were tested separately (Alleyne et al., 2010; Ambrey & Fleming, 2014; J. Li & Z. Liu, 2018). These studies are not sufficiently to reveal the way how life satisfaction is affected by various experiences in the society. Additionally, from the practical perspective, the internal migrants in China have long been regarded as an important part of China's development, but meanwhile they are facing many problems which have negative impacts on their well-being (Liu, Dijst, & Geertman, 2015). Thus, exploring ways to improve their life satisfaction is of high priority. In the present study, the results indicate that economic factors and perceived stress have similar effects on life satisfaction as previous studies, and further perceived stress can explain a part of the effects of economic factors on life satisfaction. Because only partial mediation effects of perceived stress were found, there are other potential mediators that may play important roles in explaining the relationship between economic factors and life satisfaction. Therefore, more efforts should be put into the research on life satisfaction in the future.

Consistent with Hypothesis 3, the moderating effect of social integration on the mediation effect of perceived stress linking economic factors and life satisfaction among internal migrants is significant, which suggests that the mediating effect of perceived stress in the relationship between migrants' economic factors and life satisfaction is affected by the level of social integration. With the increase of migrants' social integration, the mediating effect of perceived stress in the relationship between migrants' life satisfaction and economic factors is facilitated, while the direct effect of their economic factors on life satisfaction is relatively weakened. On the contrary, when the social integration level of the internal migrants is low, the mediating effect of perceived stress in the relationship between migrants' life satisfaction and economic factors is weakened, while the direct effect of the economic factors on life satisfaction is relatively increased. On one hand, social integration can buffer the impact of stressors on stress responses (Schwarzer et al., 2014). On the other hand, social integration itself is associated with better life satisfaction, which suggests that even stress is present, the life satisfaction is not reduced as much as that among internal migrants with lower lever of social integration (Angelini, Casi, & Corazzini, 2015).

An intervention on perceived stress is a potential way to improve life satisfaction among Chinese internal migrants. The intervention will be more effective in those with a high level of social integration. More attention should be paid to the life satisfaction of internal migrants with a relatively low level of social integration. The findings will provide new evidences advancing our understanding of the mechanism of life satisfaction among internal migrants in China, and provide support for policy makers to improve migrants' quality of life.

There is a limitation in the present study that is important to be considered. This is a cross-sectional study, so explicit causal conclusions cannot be drawn from the findings. The models in the present study need to be confirmed by longitudinal studies. Findings of this study provide data needed for further studies to verify the moderated mediation mechanisms with more rigorous longitudinal designs.

References

Alleyne, M., Alleyne, P., & Greenidge, D. (2010). Life satisfaction and perceived stress among university students in Barbados. *Journal of Psychology in Africa, 20*(2), 291–297.

Ambrey, C. L., & Fleming, C. M. (2014). The causal effect of income on life satisfaction and the implications for valuing non-market goods. *Economics Letters, 123*(2), 131–134.

Angelini, V., Casi, L., & Corazzini, L. (2015). Life satisfaction of immigrants: Does cultural assimilation matter? *Journal of Population Economics, 28*(3), 817–844.

Cohen, S., Kamarck, T., & Mermelstein, R. (1983). A global measure of perceived stress. *Journal of Health and Social Behavior, 24*(4), 385–396.

Cummins, R. A. (1996). The domains of life satisfaction: An attempt to order chaos. *Social Indicators Research, 38*(3), 303–328.

Diener, E., Inglehart, R., & Tay, L. (2013). Theory and validity of life satisfaction scales. *Social Indicators Research, 112*(3), 497–527.

Eid, M., & Larsen, R. J. (2008). *The science of subjective well-being*. New York: Guilford Press.

Eskin, M., Savk, E., Uslu, M., & Küçükaydoğan, N. (2014). Social problem-solving, perceived stress, negative life events, depression and life satisfaction in psoriasis. *Journal of the European Academy of Dermatology and Venereology, 28*(11), 1553–1559.

Extremera, N., Duran, A., & Rey, L. (2009). The moderating effect of trait meta-mood and perceived stress on life satisfaction. *Personality and Individual Differences, 47*(2), 116–121.

Gere, J., & Schimmack, U. (2017). Benefits of income: associations with life satisfaction among earners and homemakers. *Personality and Individual Differences, 119,* 92–95.

Gray, S. A., Rogers, M. A., Martinussen, R., & Tannock, R. (2015). Longitudinal relations among inattention, working memory, and academic achievement: testing mediation and the moderating role of gender. *Peer J, 3*(2), e939.

Haid, M.-L., & Seiffge-Krenke, I. (2013). Effects of (un)employment on young couples' health and life satisfaction. *Psychology & Health, 28*(3), 284–301.

Hayes, A. F. (2018). *Introduction to mediation, moderation, and conditional process analysis: a regression-based approach* (2nd ed.). New York: Guilford Press.

Herbers, D., & Mulder, C. H. (2017). Housing and subjective well-being of older adults in Europe. *Journal of Housing and the Built Environment, 32*(3), 533–558.

Hessels, J., Arampatzi, E., Der Zwan, P. V., & Burger, M. J. (2018). Life satisfaction and self-employment in different types of occupations. *Applied Economics Letters, 25*(11), 734–740.

Howell, R., & Howell, C. J. (2008). The relation of economic status to subjective well-being in developing countries: a meta-analysis. *Psychological Bulletin, 134*(4), 536–560.

Joseph, J. J., & Golden, S. H. (2017). Cortisol dysregulation: the bidirectional link between stress, depression, and type 2 diabetes mellitus. *Annals of the New York Academy of Sciences, 1391*(1), 20–34.

Kahneman, D., & Deaton, A. (2010). High income improves evaluation of life but not emotional well-being. *Proceedings of the National Academy of Sciences, 107*(38), 16489–16493.

Lazarus, R. S., & Folkman, S. (1984). *Stress, appraisal, and coping*. Springer.

Li, J., & Liu, Z. (2018a). Housing stress and mental health of migrant populations in urban China. *Cities, 81,* 172–179.

Li, J., & Liu, Z. L. (2018b). Housing stress and mental health of migrant populations in urban China. *Cities, 81,* 172–179. https://doi.org/10.1016/j.cities.2018.04.006.

Liu, Y., Dijst, M., & Geertman, S. (2015). Residential segregation and well-being inequality over time: A study on the local and migrant elderly people in Shanghai. *Cities, 49,* 1–13.

Lucas, R. E., & Dyrenforth, P. S. (2006). *Does the existence of social relationships matter for subjective well-being? Self and relationships: connecting intrapersonal and interpersonal processes*. New York: Guilford Press.

Nabi, R. L., Prestin, A., & So, J. (2013). Facebook friends with (health) benefits? Exploring social network site use and perceptions of social support, stress, and well-being. *Cyberpsychology, Behavior, and Social Networking, 16*(10), 721–727.

Pavot, W., & Diener, E. (1993). Review of the satisfaction with life scale. *Psychological Assessment, 5*(2), 164–172.

Pavot, W., & Diener, E. (2009). Review of the satisfaction with life scale. In E. Diener (Ed.), *Assessing well-being: the collected works of Ed Diener*. Dordrecht: Springer Netherlands.

Rey, L., & Extremera, N. (2015). Core self-evaluations, perceived stress and life satisfaction in Spanish young and middle-aged adults: An examination of mediation and moderation effects. *Social Indicators Research, 120*(2), 515–524.

Rossi, N., & Bisconti, T. (2003). The meditational effect of hardiness on perceived stress and life satisfaction following conjugal loss. *Gerontologist, 43*(S1), 199.

Rupert, M. S., & Hawi, N. (2016). Relationships among smartphone addiction, stress, academic performance, and satisfaction with life. *Computers in Human Behavior, 57,* 321–325.

Sanders, F., & Maria, A. (2014). *Life satisfaction, social identity, and household work: An intersectionality perspective*, (Doctor of Philosophy). University of Memphis (3648489).

Schwarzer, R., Bowler, R. M., & Cone, J. E. (2014). Social integration buffers stress in New York police after the 9/11 terrorist attack. *Anxiety Stress and Coping, 27*(1), 18–26.

Sehlen, S., Vordermark, D., Schäfer, C., Herschbach, P., Bayerl, A., Pigorsch, S., et al. (2009). Job stress and job satisfaction of physicians, radiographers, nurses and physicists working in radiotherapy: a multicenter analysis by the DEGRO Quality of Life Work Group. *Radiation Oncology, 4*(1), e6.

Shi, M., Wang, X., Bian, Y., & Wang, L. (2015). The mediating role of resilience in the relationship between stress and life satisfaction among Chinese medical students: a cross-sectional study. *BMC Medical Education, 15*(1), e16.

Tang, D. (2015). Social integration scale of migrant population: based on Monitoring Survey of Migrant Population 2013. *Population & Economics*(5), 25–30.

Turner, B., & Turner, J. R. (2013). *Social relations, social integration, and social support Handbook of the sociology of mental health.* Dordrecht: Springer.

Turpin, H., Urben, S., Ansermet, F., Borghini, A., Murray, M. M., & Muller-Nix, C. I. (2019). The interplay between prematurity, maternal stress and children's intelligence quotient at age 11: A longitudinal study. *Scientific Reports, 9*(1), e450.

Tuyen, T. Q., & Vu, H. V. (2018). A microeconometric analysis of housing and life satisfaction among the Vietnamese elderly. *Quality & Quantity, 52*(2), 849–867.

Wang, K. T., Yuen, M., & Slaney, R. B. (2008). Perfectionism, depression, loneliness, and life satisfaction: a study of high school students in Hong Kong. *The Counseling Psychologist, 37*(2), 249–274.

Wiegner, L., Hange, D., Björkelund, C., & Ahlborg, G. (2015). Prevalence of perceived stress and associations to symptoms of exhaustion, depression and anxiety in a working age population seeking primary care-an observational study. *BMC Family Practice, 16*(1), e38.

Yoo, C. M. (2016). Does perceived social support moderate the effects of care giving stress on life satisfaction of siblings of people with intellectual disabilities in South Korea? *Journal of Intellectual Disability Research, 60*(7–8), 821.

Zhang, F., Zhang, C., & Hudson, J. (2018). Housing conditions and life satisfaction in urban China. *Cities, 81,* 35–44.

Zhou, Z.-K., Liu, Q.-Q., Niu, G.-F., Sun, X.-J., & Fan, C.-Y. (2017). Bullying victimization and depression in Chinese children: a moderated mediation model of resilience and mindfulness. *Personality and Individual Differences, 104,* 137–142.

Chapter 7
Effects of Migration Experiences on the Health of Internal Migrants

Chaoping Pan

1 Introduction

Population migration, including domestic and international migration, is an objective phenomenon in the process of globalization and urbanization. And the global migratory crisis also witnesses unprecedented numbers of people on the move and tremendous diversity in terms of age, gender and medical requirements (Abbas et al., 2018). And they have varying degrees of vulnerability and needs in terms of protection, security, rights, and access to healthcare. Report on China's Migrant Population Development 2018 shows that the total number of internal migrants in China reached 245 million in 2017. With the rapid development of industry in China, Chinese internal migrants may also have varies of health problems, such as chronic diseases, occupational diseases, venereal diseases and so on, which are caused by complex reasons such as diversity health needs of migrants and imperfect health care system. Migrants' health need and its diversity also attract the attention of Chinese government (Mou, Griffiths, Fong, & Dawes, 2015).

Migrants always lack basic health care, public health services and medical insurance because they do not have local resident registration (*hukou*) in the place where they migrated. Although the central government has put forward some strategies such as "Healthy China 2020" and "Healthy China 2030", as well as some policies such as "settlement of medical insurance in different places" and "equalization of basic public health services of internal migrants", the implementation of these policies still needs to be strengthened. The "Healthy China 2030" strategy attaches great importance to social determines of health, and proposes to carry out precise health interventions. However, in internal migrants, how to provide precise services should consider how migration process affects the health of them.

C. Pan (✉)
School of Health Sciences, Wuhan University, Wuhan, China
e-mail: 2019103050012@whu.edu.cn

P. Wang (ed.), *The Health Status of Internal Migrants in China*,
https://doi.org/10.1007/978-981-15-4415-6_7

The process of migration is a series of events constituted by a number of factors over a period of time, and it can be divided into four stages: pre-migration stage, migration stage, detention stage and return stage, and migrants' health is more probably to change during migration and retention stages (Hollander et al., 2019). For example, the migration stage may increase the risks of infectious diseases, motion sickness, traffic accidents and the pressure of migration in travellers visiting friends and relatives and in sexual encounters away from home (Fricker & Steffen, 2008); and the health of internal migrants in detention stage may be influenced by occupational health, social support and integration, health security and health service accessibility, etc. (Bonmati-Tomas et al., 2019; Li, Sun, Li, & Durkin, 2019; Rask et al., 2018; Staniforth & Such, 2019). Migration experiences during the migration and detention stages are the key determinants of migrants' health (Bhugra, 2004).

Plenty of studies have shown that migration experiences have different impacts on the health of different migrant populations, as well as the health between migrants and non-migrants (Mou et al., 2015; Villa & Raviglione, 2019). Trilesnik et al. found that ex-soviet jews are significantly more depressed and more anxious than native Austrians but are less likely to be affected by clinical depression (Trilesnik, Koch, & Stompe, 2018). Gkiouleka et al. discovered that migrants have more depressive symptoms in seven of the examined countries, while in Greece and the UK, they have less depressive symptoms compared with non-migrant population (Gkiouleka et al., 2018). Tong et al. found a health disadvantage in the elderly who had ever migrated. However, the age-health profile of rural ever-migrants is not different from that of rural non-migrants (Tong, Piotrowski, & Ye, 2018).

Prior researches have also studied group disparities of the effect of migration on migrants' health. Ivanova et al. found that female migrants are more vulnerable to poor self-rated health (SRH) outcomes and their knowledge regarding contraceptive methods, STIs and HIV/AIDS are limited (Ivanova, Rai, & Kemigisha, 2018). Ebrahim et al. found that rural men have lower blood pressure, lipids, and fasting blood glucose than urban and migrant men and no differences are found in women (Ebrahim et al., 2010). Long et al. found that the initial health advantage among Chinese rural-to-urban migrant workers is largely due to self-selection rather than migration effects, and this will exacerbate the contradiction between the allocation of medical resources and the demand in rural and urban China (Long, Han, & Liu, 2020).

However, previous researches also have the following limitations. First, plenty of studies focus on the disparities in health between migrants and non-migrants, but few empirical researches pay attention to the internal disparities caused by migration experiences of migrants especially in the social context of China (Aarabi et al., 2018; Kuhn, Barham, Razzaque, & Turner, 2020; Ma et al., 2020); second, most previous studies analyze the health effects of internal migration by general or generalized linear regression analysis, which cannot control the selection bias well and yield a biased estimation (Long et al., 2020; Reus-Pons, Mulder, Kibele, & Janssen, 2018); third, most studies use regional, not nationwide database, which restrains the national representativeness of them (Lommel, Hu, Sun, & Chen, 2020).

2 Data and Methods

2.1 Data Source and Key Variables

The data used in this chapter were from the China Migrants Dynamic Survey (CMDS) in 2018. A stratified, multi-stage and probability proportionate to size (PPS) method was used in CMDS 2018 to ensure the representativeness of the sample. A total of 170,000 migrants were surveyed and used in this study. Self-rated health (SRH) was used as the dependent variable, migrating experiences including migration duration and migrating to other cities ever before were used as independent variables, and some personal characteristics (age, gender, education, work status, family income, *hukou*), awareness rate of basic public health services, community characteristics and regional economic level were used as control variables.

2.2 Econometric Models

In this chapter, the effects of migration experiences on SRH of internal migrants were examined using Propensity Score Matching (PSM) approach. Groups of migration duration with 10 years or more and migrating to other cities ever before were as treatment groups; migration duration with 10 year and below and never migrating to other cities ever before were considered as control groups. Subsequently, PSM was operated to calculate the average treatment effects on the treated (ATT) in different groups. With other covariates controlled for, the conditional probability of different groups of internal migrants was estimated, and the model was as follows:

$$\ln\left(\frac{p_i}{1-p_i}\right) = \alpha + \sum_{t=1_t}^{T} \beta_t x_{it} + i\varepsilon_i$$

where $p_i = P(T_i = 1|X_{it})$ represented the probability that the internal migrants belonged to treatment group. The matched mean values of SRH between control and treatment groups were compared to find out the effects of two specific treatments (Migration duration of 10 years or more, and migrating to other cities ever before) on the health of internal migrants.

$$\text{ATT} = \frac{1}{N_1} \sum_{i:D_i=1} (y_i - \bar{y}_{0i}) = \frac{1}{N_1} \sum_{i:D_i=1} \left(y_i - \sum_{j:D_j=1} w(i, j) y_j \right)$$

where $N_1 = \sum_i D_i$ was the number of treatment groups, and y_i was the SRH of treatment groups, $w(i, j)$ were the weights of (i, j) and y_j were the SRH of matched groups. The different matching methods were mainly reflected in the weights of $w(i, j)$.

3 Results

3.1 Basic Information

The mean value of SRH was 3.79 and most of the migrants reported to be healthy or basically healthy, indicating a good health status of internal migrants. The mean value of migration duration and migrating to other cities ever before were 0.22 and 0.47, respectively, indicating that 78% internal migrants stayed in local area less than 10 years in this migration and 53% of them had never migrated to other cities ever before. Most internal migrants were young adults, and the mean age was 37.55 years old; males account for 52% of the respondents and were slightly more than females; most internal migrants had a low education level, and the mean value was only 1.57; a total of 18% internal migrants was unemployed; the average household income was 1.73, indicating that most internal migrants lived in a family with a low level of family income; a total of 83% internal migrants had agricultural *hukou*; most internal migrants had a spouse, but there was still 18% having no spouse.

For community characteristics, most migrants were close to the community health service center, with a distance less than 30 min; most migrants (73%) lived in neighborhood committees. A total of 40% migrants had never heard of basic public health services, and the average type of health education received was 3.75. The majority of internal migrants (83%) had a willingness of long-term residence. The average value of the illness within one year was 2.45, indicating most internal migrants did not develop disease within recent two weeks. Most of internal migrants lived in high economic region and medium economic region, and less of them lived in a poor economic region. More details can be seen in Table 1.

3.2 Group Disparities in the Relationship Between Migration Experiences and SRH: Based on Ordinary Least Squares (OLS)

With other variables controlled for, there was a significant relationship between migration experiences and SRH, and some significant group disparities were also observed. First, an educational disparity was found, and a longer duration of migration was significantly related to poorer SRH ($\beta = -0.030$, $p < 0.001$) only in migrants receiving junior high school education or below; migrating to other cities ever before significantly related to poorer SHR and negative SHR effects was more obvious in senior high school group. Second, a gender disparity was observed;

Table 1 Basic information of variables used

Variables	Mean	SD	Min	Max	Variable coding
Dependent variable					
SRH	3.79	0.47	1	4	1 = disability, 2 = unhealthy, 3 = basic health, 4 = health
Independent variables					
Migrating time	0.22	0.41	0	1	0 = 0–10 years, 1 = 10 years or longer
Migrating to other cities ever before	0.47	0.50	0	1	0 = no, 1 = yes
Control variables					
Age	37.55	11.08	16.09	97.39	Continuous variable
Male	0.52	0.50	0	1	0 = female, 1 = male
Education	1.57	0.77	1	3	1 = junior high school or below, 2 = senior high school, 3 = college or above
Having a job	0.82	0.38	0	1	0 = no job, 1 = having job
Family income	1.73	0.55	1	3	1 = low income, 2 = middle income income, 3 = high income
Non-agricultural	0.17	0.38	0	1	0 = agricultural, 1 = non-agricultural
Having spouse	0.82	0.38	0	1	0 = no spouse, 1 = having a spouse
Distance to community health service center	1.19	0.45	1	4	1 = 15 min or less, 2 = between 15–30 min, 3 = between 0.5–1 h, 4 = 1 h or more
Village committee	0.27	0.44	0	1	0 = neighborhood committee, 1 = village committee
Regional economic level	1.91	0.88	1	3	1 = high level, 2 = middle level, 3 = low level
Willingness of long-term residence	0.83	0.38	0	1	0 = not willing/clear, 1 = willing to live
Knowing the national basic public health service	0.60	0.49	0	1	0 = not know, 1 = know
Accepting health education	3.75	3.39	0	9	Continuous variable
Illness within one year	2.45	0.61	1	3	1 = illness within two week, 2 = illness within one year, 3 = no illness within one year

Note SD: standard deviation

migrating to other cities ever before would have a stronger negative association with male's SRH than with female's (for males, $\beta = -0.025, p < 0.001$; for females, $\beta = -0.012, p < 0.001$); but a longer duration of migration would have a stronger negative association to female's SRH than male's (for males, $\beta = -0.019, p < 0.001$; for females, $\beta = -0.023, p < 0.001$).

Third, a family income disparity was also observed; living in a local area for more than 10 years had a stronger negative association with SRH in internal migrants with low-level family income than with middle- or high-level family income ($\beta = -0.050$, $p < 0.001$ for low family income; $\beta = -0.008, p < 0.05$ for middle family income; $\beta = -0.018, p > 0.05$ for high family income); migrating to other cities ever before had a stronger negative association with SRH in migrants with middle-level family income than in migrants with low- or high-level family income migrants ($\beta = -0.005, p > 0.05$ for low family income; $\beta = -0.024, p < 0.001$ for middle family income; $\beta = -0.014, p > 0.05$ for high family income). Finally, the type of *hukou* also mattered; although migrating more than one time was related to poorer SRH in migrants with both type of *hukou*, a longer duration of migration was significantly related to poorer SRH ($\beta = -0.023, p < 0.001$) only in migrants with an agricultural *hukou*. See Table 2.

Table 2 Group disparities in the relationship between migration experiences and SRH: based on OLS

Groups	Junior school and below	Senior high school	College or above	Male	Female
Migrating time	−0.030***	−0.012	−0.010	−0.019***	−0.023***
Migrating to other cities ever before	−0.017***	−0.021***	−0.019***	−0.025***	−0.012***
	Low-level family income	Middle-level family income	High-level family income	Non-agricultural	Agricultural
Migration duration	−0.050***	−0.008*	−0.018	−0.010	−0.023***
Migrating to other cities ever before	−0.005	−0.024***	−0.014	−0.024***	−0.016***

Note $^{*}p < 0.05$, $^{**}p < 0.01$, $^{***}p < 0.001$. The control variables were age, male, education, work status, family income, *hukou*, having spouse, distance to community health service center, type of committee, regional economic level, willingness of long-term residence, knowledge of national basic public health services, types of health education received, and illness within one year; the number in the table was the coefficient of OLS models

3.3 Group Disparities in the Relationship Between Migration Experiences and SRH: Based on PSM

Table 3 showed that, both Pseudo R2 and LR CHI2 decreased significantly in all sub-groups; except for the female and agricultural population, the total bias of all the other sub-groups were not significant at 0.05 levels, which meant selection bias was basically controlled for after PSM.

The results of nearest neighbor matching (1:4) showed that the longer migration duration was related to poorer SRH but only significant in junior school and bellow and senior high school groups (for junior school and bellow, ATT = −0.038, $p < 0.001$; for senior high school, ATT = −0.020, $p < 0.01$; for college or above, ATT = 0.002, $p > 0.05$). Migrating to other cities ever before was associated with a poorer SRH but only significant in junior school and bellow and senior high school groups (for junior school and bellow, ATT = −0.021, $p < 0.001$; for senior high school, ATT = −0.019, $p < 0.001$; for college or above, ATT = −0.019, $p > 0.05$). In terms of household income, the longer migration duration was significantly related to a poorer SRH but only significant in low- and middle-income families (for low-income families, ATT = −0.061, $p < 0.001$; for middle-income families, ATT = −0.016, $p < 0.001$; for high-income families, ATT = 0.021, $p > 0.05$) and migrating to other cities ever before was associated with poorer SRH but only significant in middle-level family income (for low-level family income, ATT = −0.005, $p > 0.05$; for middle-level family income, ATT = −0.026, $p < 0.001$; for high-level family income, ATT = −0.013, $p > 0.05$).

As for *hukou*, the longer migration duration associated with poorer SRH but only significant in groups with agricultural *hukou* (for agricultural, ATT = −0.034, $p < 0.001$; for non-agricultural, ATT = −0.014, $p > 0.05$); migrating to other cities ever before was significantly associated with poorer SRH in groups with both non-agricultural and agricultural *hukou*, but the association was more stronger in non-agricultural migrants (for non-agricultural, ATT = −0.024, $p < 0.001$; for Agricultural, ATT = −0.019, $p < 0.001$). In terms of gender, a longer migration duration was significantly associated with poorer SRH in both sexes, but it was stronger in the female group (for female, ATT = −0.042, $p < 0.001$; for male, ATT = −0.028, $p < 0.001$); migrating to other cities ever before was significantly related with poorer SRH both in both sexes, and the association was stronger in males (for female, ATT = −0.012, $p < 0.001$; for male, ATT = −0.024, $p < 0.001$). See Table 4.

Caliper matching was operated for sensitivity analysis and OLS regression was used to illustrate the effects of PSM. The results of caliper matching were basically consistent with that of nearest neighbor matching (1:4), which showed a robust estimation of PSM. Compared with OLS regression, the results of PSM showed that the association between SHR and migration experiences was stronger. Therefore, using OLS regression may underestimate the association between migration experiences and internal migrants' health.

Table 3 Selection bias of control variables before and after matching

Groups		Migration duration		Migrating to other cities ever before	
nearest neighbor matching (1:4)		Pseudo R2	LR chi2	Pseudo R2	LR chi2
junior school or bellow	Before match	0.081	8933.14***	0.065	8351.07***
	After match	0.000	19.63	0.000	10.16
Senior high school	Before match	0.101	3465.79***	0.060	2804.79***
	After match	0.000	9.56	0.000	5.64
College or above	Before match	0.115	2605.82***	0.045	1688.07***
	After match	0.002	21.66	0.000	10.23
Low-level family income	Before match	0.121	6550.22***	0.047	3048.01***
	After match	0.000	11.21	0.000	4.72
Middle-level family income	Before match	0.091	9571.59***	0.051	6884.45***
	After match	0.000	13.66	0.000	7.66
High-level family income	Before match	0.081	804.10***	0.058	649.84***
	After match	0.002	14.82	0.000	5.72
Non-agricultural	Before match	0.078	2286.61***	0.060	2206.91***
	After match	0.001	10.59	0.000	7.43
Agricultural	Before match	0.103	14443.58***	0.061	10669.40***
	After match	0.000	37.62***	0.000	11.56
Female	Before match	0.106	8285.00***	0.056	5706.36***
	After match	0.001	38.22***	0.000	11.21
Male	Before match	0.090	8138.82***	0.056	6226.43***
	After match	0.001	22.95	0.000	16.23

Note $^{*}p < 0.05$, $^{**}p < 0.01$, $^{***}p < 0.001$

Table 4 Group disparities in the relationship between migration experiences and SRH: based on PSM

Groups		Migration duration		Migrating to other cities ever before	
		ATT	SE	ATT	SE
Junior school or below	Nearest neighbor matching (1:4)	−0.038***	0.005	−0.021***	0.004
	Caliper matching	−0.032***	0.006	−0.018***	0.005
Senior high school	Nearest neighbor matching (1:4)	−0.020**	0.007	−0.019***	0.005
	Caliper matching	−0.014	0.009	−0.017**	0.006
College or above	Nearest neighbor matching (1:4)	0.002	0.008	−0.019***	0.005
	Caliper matching	0.0001	0.009	−0.022***	0.006
Low-level family income	Nearest neighbor matching (1:4)	−0.061***	0.008	−0.005	0.006
	Caliper matching	−0.059***	0.010	−0.009	0.007
Middle-level family income	Nearest neighbor matching (1:4)	−0.016***	0.004	−0.026***	0.003
	Caliper matching	−0.016**	0.005	−0.027***	0.004
High-level family income	Nearest neighbor matching (1:4)	0.021	0.011	−0.013	0.010
	Caliper matching	0.024	0.014	−0.022	0.011
Non-agricultural	Nearest neighbor matching (1:4)	−0.014	0.009	−0.024**	0.007
	Caliper matching	−0.014	0.011	−0.025**	0.008
Agricultural	Nearest neighbor matching (1:4)	−0.034***	0.004	−0.019***	0.003
	Caliper matching	−0.039***	0.005	−0.018***	0.003
Female	Nearest neighbor matching (1:4)	−0.042***	0.006	−0.012**	0.004
	Caliper matching	−0.047***	0.007	−0.015**	0.005
Male	Nearest neighbor matching (1:4)	−0.028***	0.005	−0.024***	0.004
	Caliper matching	−0.033***	0.006	−0.025***	0.004

Note $^{*}p < 0.05$, $^{**}p < 0.01$, $^{***}p < 0.001$. ATT: Average Treatment Effect on the Treated. SE: standard error

4 Discussion and Suggestions

The results of this chapter showed that Chinese internal migrants had a good SRH status overall with a low one-year prevalence rate. Those were in line with the health selection phenomenon at the beginning of migration, that is, healthier people are more likely to migrate and become migrants. A total of 47% internal migrants had ever migrated to other cities, and most migrants had stayed in local area no more than 10 years, indicating that most Chinese internal migrants have a short-term migration experiences and were hard to have a stable work.

Although most internal migrants had jobs, they had received less education, earn less income and had a low occupational status. Most internal migrants were rural-to-urban migrants and had an agricultural *hukou*, which may be a barrier for their social integration in local area. Although most migrants lived in neighborhood committees and could reach community healthcare centers within 15 min (a better geographical access to health services), they received less health education and had low-level health awareness, which may be due to the common phenomenon of "emphasizing medical treatment and neglecting prevention" and is not conducive to their health (Lu & Qin, 2014).

The results of PSM showed that migration duration and migrating to other cities ever before were both associated with the health of internal migrants, and the associations were different among different sub-groups. The longer migration duration had an association with poorer SRH of internal migrants only in groups with junior high school or below group, and had non-association in groups with senior high school level or above education; the SRH of migrants with more education and high-level family income had non-association with migration duration, this may be related to a better employment environment, more health resources and better health education.

The longer migration duration had association with poorer health status of internal migrants with agricultural *hukou*, rather than non-agricultural internal migrants. This may be caused by two reasons. First, the "farming" life pattern is quite different from the life in modern cities, and rural-to-urban migrants have a relatively poor adaption to urban consumption and lifestyle, which may lead to a greater loss of health due to a longer migrating duration. Second, the results showed that the non-agricultural internal migrants often possessed higher education level, so they may also have higher health education (Salazar & Hu, 2016).

In terms of gender, longer migration duration had a significant association with poorer SRH, but it was stronger in women migrants than that in males (Kuhn et al., 2020). This may be due to two reasons: first, women are burdened with both housework and child care, this may increase the health costs during their migration; second, women's work is limited by childcare and other constraints, so they tend to accept a low-paid job, which may limit their investment in health (Xie & Cen, 2019).

The results showed that migrating to other cities ever before had an association with poorer health in groups with middle-level family only. Because migtants with low-level family income have stronger resistance to migration in migration stage; while migrants with middle- and high-level income have more incomes, health education, social capital and more resources available to address harmful factors encountered during migration.

Migrating to other cities ever before was associated with poorer SRH of internal migrants and it was stronger in groups with non-agricultural *hukou*, probably because migrants with agricultural *hukou* have a greater adaptability to migration and less health loss. Migrating to other cities ever before was related to migrant's poorer SRH and it was stronger in males than that in females. As family-based migration is rising among internal migrants in China, female migrants are more likely to migrate as spouses and family members, so male migrants are traditionally more likely to undertake responsibilities during the travels and when living in an unfamiliar place, which may lead to a greater toll on men's health.

The policy supports are important to reduce the health deterioration of migrants. Migrants will have less health problems and health care access barriers in countries that have more health policies for migrants than those having less (Reyes-Uruena, Noori, Pharris, & Jansa, 2014). Thus, it is necessary to provide more health services and reallocate the health resources effectively to meet different health needs of migrants. The results showed that migrates may have a low health knowledge level that lead to more serious health deterioration, so they required more health education to develop scientific healthcare-seeking behaviors. However, health education for migrants is still weak in China. It is proposed the government should strengthen health education for internal migrants and provide precise services for internal migrants with different health needs in the future (Li, Yang, Wang, & Liu, 2020).

Migrants had frequent movements which would increase the degree of health deterioration during their migration and were greater for men than for women in China. Therefore, it is suggested to strengthen health protection in migration stage, such as environmental sanitation and public facility improvement of train and bus station, implementing health education for internal migrants (especially the male) to improve their health prevention ability and so on (Korzeniewski, 2017).

Migrants also earned less than social average, so they had fewer resources to invest on their health. Therefore, it is suggested that inter-region medical insurance settlement process should be strengthened to reduce the burden of diseases of internal migrants and the labor remuneration of internal migrants should be raised by improving social minimum wage level (Lu, Qian, & Ma, 2013). Internal migrants with less income level and agricultural *hukou* may have a serious health deterioration caused by poor employment environment and insufficient health resources. Therefore, it is suggested to improve the relative laws and regulations and focus on improving the working environment of migrants with less education, less income level and agricultural *hukou*.

Short migration duration may cause poor SRH as a result of a low social integration, or even discrimination from local residents. It is, therefore, recommended to encourage migrants to actively participate in local social activities to reduce social isolation and improve health. As female migrants may experience more serious health loss due to a longer retention, it is recommended to avoid employment discrimination, provide more inclusive employment environment for female migrants and avoid adverse pregnancy outcomes to improve their health level by combining the institutional, national and local public health actions. Migrants with middle-level family income and non-agricultural *hukou* may be more fragile to suffer from health damages to health damages when they want to earn more money. Therefore, it is recommended to pay more attention to the health of them for the purpose of health equity, enhance their ability to deal with migration pressure and reduce health deterioration by strengthening their health education.

This chapter makes the following important contributions. First, as migrants' health is an urgent problem in worldwide, the paper focused on group disparities in the impacts of migration experiences on migrants' health which can help the government and people better understand the effects of migration experiences on different migrants' health. According to the results, the government should issue policies precisely to improve the health of different migrants and the efficiency of health resource allocation. Second, we used a causal inference method PSM, which can have a better control of the selection bias than other common methods. However, as we use a cross-sectional survey and use a single self-rated health indicator, the results still need to be further proved using longitudinal researches and more complicated indicators in the future.

References

Aarabi, G., Reissmann, D. R., Sagheri, D., Neuschulz, J., Heydecke, G., Kofahl, C., et al. (2018). Oral health-related quality of life of children and adolescents with and without migration background in Germany. *Quality of Life Research, 27*(10), 2619–2627.

Abbas, M., Aloudat, T., Bartolomei, J., Carballo, M., Durieux-Paillard, S., Gabus, L., et al. (2018). Migrant and refugee populations: a public health and policy perspective on a continuing global crisis. *Antimicrobial Resistance and Infection Control, 7,* 113.

Bhugra, D. (2004). Migration and mental health. *Acta Psychiatrica Scand, 109*(4), 243–258.

Bonmati-Tomas, A., Malagon-Aguilera, M. C., Gelabert-Vilella, S., Bosch-Farre, C., Vaandrager, L., Garcia-Gil, M. M., et al. (2019). Salutogenic health promotion program for migrant women at risk of social exclusion. *International Journal for Equity in Health, 18*(1), 139.

Ebrahim, S., Kinra, S., Bowen, L., Andersen, E., Ben-Shlomo, Y., Lyngdoh, T., et al. (2010). The effect of rural-to-urban migration on obesity and diabetes in India: a cross-sectional study. *PLoS Medicine, 7*(4), e1000268.

Fricker, M., & Steffen, R. (2008). Travel and public health. *Journal of Infect Public Health, 1*(2), 72–77.

Gkiouleka, A., Avrami, L., Kostaki, A., Huijts, T., Eikemo, T. A., & Stathopoulou, T. (2018). Depressive symptoms among migrants and non-migrants in Europe: documenting and explaining inequalities in times of socio-economic instability. *European Journal of Public Health, 28*(suppl_5), 54–60.

Hollander, A. C., Pitman, A., Sjoqvist, H., Lewis, G., Magnusson, C., Kirkbride, J. B., & Dalman, C. (2019). Suicide risk among refugees compared with non-refugee migrants and the Swedish-born majority population. *The British Journal of Psychiatry*, 1–7.

Ivanova, O., Rai, M., & Kemigisha, E. (2018). A systematic review of sexual and reproductive health knowledge, experiences and access to services among refugee, migrant and displaced girls and young women in Africa. *International Journal of Environmental Research and Public Health, 15*(8), 1583.

Korzeniewski, K. (2017). Travel health prevention. *Internation Maritime Health, 68*(4), 238–244.

Kuhn, R., Barham, T., Razzaque, A., & Turner, P. (2020). Health and well-being of male international migrants and non-migrants in Bangladesh: A cross-sectional follow-up study. *PLoS Medicine, 17*(3), e1003081.
Li, W., Sun, F., Li, Y., & Durkin, D. W. (2019). Work stress and depressive symptoms in chinese migrant workers: The moderating role of community factors. *Journal of Immigrant and Minority Health, 21*(6), 1248–1256.
Li, X., Yang, H., Wang, H., & Liu, X. (2020). Effect of health education on healthcare-seeking behavior of migrant workers in China. *International Journal of Environmental Reserch and Public Health, 17*(7), 2344.
Lommel, L., Hu, X., Sun, M., & Chen, J. L. (2020). Frequency of depressive symptoms among female migrant workers in China: Associations with acculturation, discrimination, and reproductive health. *Public Health, 181,* 151–157.
Long, C., Han, J., & Liu, Y. (2020). Has rural-urban migration promoted the health of chinese migrant workers? *International Journal of Environmental Research and Public Health, 17*(4), 1218.
Lu, H., Qian, W., & Ma, Z. (2013). Study on labor supply behaviors of the women of rural migrant households. *Statistics & Information Forum, 28*(9), 100–106.
Lu, Y., & Qin, L. (2014). Healthy migrant and salmon bias hypotheses: A study of health and internal migration in China. *Social Science and Medicine, 102,* 41–48.
Ma, S., Li, Q., Zhou, X., Cao, W., Jiang, M., & Li, L. (2020). Assessment of health inequality between urban-to-urban and rural-to-urban migrant older adults in China: a cross-sectional study. *BMC Public Health, 20*(1), 268.
Mou, J., Griffiths, S. M., Fong, H. F., & Dawes, M. G. (2015). Defining migration and its health impact in China. *Public Health, 129*(10), 1326–1334.
Rask, S., Elo, I. T., Koskinen, S., Lilja, E., Koponen, P., & Castaneda, A. E. (2018). The association between discrimination and health: Findings on Russian, Somali and Kurdish origin populations in Finland. *European Journal of Public Health, 28*(5), 898–903.
Reus-Pons, M., Mulder, C. H., Kibele, E. U. B., & Janssen, F. (2018). Differences in the health transition patterns of migrants and non-migrants aged 50 and older in southern and western Europe (2004–2015). *BMC Medicine, 16*(1), 57.
Reyes-Uruena, J. M., Noori, T., Pharris, A., & Jansa, J. M. (2014). New times for migrants' health in Europe. *Revista Espanola De Sanidad Penitenciaria, 16*(2), 48–58.
Salazar, M. A., & Hu, X. (2016). Health and lifestyle changes among migrant workers in China: Implications for the healthy migrant effect. *The Lancet Diabetes & Endocrinology, 4*(2), 89–90.
Staniforth, R., & Such, E. (2019). Public health practitioners' perspectives of migrant health in an English region. *Public Health, 175,* 79–86.
Tong, Y., Piotrowski, M., & Ye, H. (2018). Differences in the health-age profile across rural and urban sectors: A study on migrants and non-migrants in China. *Public Health, 158,* 124–134.
Trilesnik, B., Koch, S. C., & Stompe, T. (2018). Mental health, acculturation and religiosity in Jewish migrants from the former Soviet Union in Austria. *Neuropsychiatrie, 32*(2), 84–92.
Villa, S., & Raviglione, M. C. (2019). Migrants' health: Building migrant-sensitive health systems. *Journal of Public Health Research, 8*(1), 1592.
Xie, P., & Cen, X. (2019). The Influence of Children's follow-up on the employment of female migrants. *Human Resources Development of China, 36*(7), 106–120.

Chapter 8
Marriage and Childbirth Situation of Internal Migrants at Different Birth Cohorts

Yuehui Wang, Hong Yan, and Jingjing Li

1 Introduction

After China's social economic reform in the later 1970s, massive labor forces' migration and re-location, mainly from rural to urban China, are caused by multiple factors, including increased economic freedom and regional disequilibrium (Zheng & Yang, 2016; Zhu, 2002). According to a recent report published by the National Bureau of Statistics of China, there is a steady growth of Chinese internal migrants, which increased from 121 million in 2000 to 253 million in 2014. Although the total number of internal migrants has slightly declined for the first time after 2015, they still account for a large proportion of the total population in China (National Bureau of Statistics, 2018).

Marriage and childbirth are two important life events (Webster & Mawer, 1989), which are influenced by personal characteristics, life experiences, religious beliefs, social networks, social background, and so on (Addo, 2014; Allendorf & Pandian, 2016; Boulier & Rosenzweig, 1978; Islam & Ahmed, 1998; Manglos-Weber & Weinreb, 2017; Patravali & Gaonkar, 1991; Rosenwalke, 1972). As a personal life experience, migration has an effect on migrants' marriage and childbirth. Carlson (1985) found that migration may delay the age of marriage and childbearing. Migration also influences the number of newborns, because migration usually disrupts the status of marital relations, resulting in the separation of spouses as well as a lower probability of childbearing (Chen, Liu, Vikram, & Guo, 2015; Rundquist & Brown, 1989). Moreover, migration may also facilitate unplanned births (Blayo, 1993). It is worth noting that migrants at different birth cohorts have quite different characteristics and

Y. Wang · H. Yan (✉)
School of Health Sciences, Wuhan University, Wuhan, China
e-mail: yanhmjxr@whu.edu.cn

J. Li
Behavioral Sciences and Health Education, Rollins School of Public Health, Emory University, Atlanta, USA

P. Wang (ed.), *The Health Status of Internal Migrants in China*,
https://doi.org/10.1007/978-981-15-4415-6_8

behavioral patterns. For example, compared with older migrants, migrant workers born latter have received more education, and more of them become white-collar workers (Zheng, 2013). The culture and behaviors related to marriage and childbirth have changed over time in different migrants, so migrants at different birth cohorts may show different marital and childbirth characteristics.

Because of the One-Child Policy, Chinese total fertility rate is lower than the normal replacement level (Goodkind, 2017; Jiang, Feldman, & Li, 2014a; Jiang, Li, & Sánchez-Barricarte, 2014b), so marriage and fertility status should be paid much attention to. For marriage and childbirth situation, age of first marriage, age of first birth and first birth interval can be used as key indicators to predict population replacement and growth (Nguyen, Nguyen, Swenson, & Pham, 1993). The age of first birth partly determines the intergenerational interval of population reproduction. An earlier first childbirth in a family usually leads to a shorter intergenerational interval and a higher generation replacement level. The combination of first birth interval and first marriage age also has an effect on population replacement and growth. If first marriage age is constant, the longer the first birth interval is, the slower the population growth will be (Nath, Singh, Land, & Talukdar, 1993; Zheng, 2000). In addition, as the interval between first birth and marriage is hardly affected by the national family planning policy (Shayan, Ayatollahi, Zare, & Moradi, 2014), first birth interval may be useful to guide the future reproductive plan for internal migrants. Generally, a shorter interval between female marriage and childbirth usually leads to a higher probability of reproduction and a higher probability of multiple children (Nenko & Jasienska, 2013).

In recent years, the scale of inter-provincial marriage among internal migrants has continuously increased with the large-scale migration in China (Wang, 2013). Compared with intra-provincial marriage, inter-provincial marriage inevitably leads to a series of problems. On the one hand, individuals with inter-provincial intermarriage have to face more problems of social cohesion. On the other hand, low costs for divorce and lack of social support lead to a poor stability of inter-provincial marriage. Furthermore, there are also problems of puppy love, early marriage and premarital pregnancy in inter-provincial marriages (Song, Zhang, & Duan, 2012).

Sexual intercourse behavior before marriage is common among Chinese internal migrants (Qi, Bao, Zhang, Yu, & Liu, 2017; Wang et al., 2013). It is estimated that there are about 10 million abortions per year in China, of which 1/3 are non-first-time abortions and most cases are rural-to-urban migrants (He et al., 2012). Using data from Shenzhen, Guangzhou and Wuhan in China, Liu et al. (2011) found that around 21% of the unmarried rural-to-urban migrants had premarital sexual experiences, and nearly half of them (47.4%) had never used condom during their sexual intercourses. Based on a survey of 944 unmarried rural-to-urban female migrants in Shanghai, China, Wang et al. (2013) found that the premarital sex and pregnancy rate of the respondents were 28.2% and 5.2%, respectively. Based on the China Migrants Dynamic Survey (CMDS) in 2013, Qi and Yang (2015) found that the proportion of unmarried pregnant couples accounted for 30.5% in migrant couples who were at first marriage and had one child.

Prior studies on the marital and childbirth situation of Chinese internal migrants are mainly based on small samples (Cai et al., 2013). Nationally representative and large sample data are less frequently used in studies on marital and childbirth situation of migrants. In this study, a comprehensive analysis on marital status, relationship between first marriage and migration, intermarriage circle, age at first marriage, age at first childbearing, first birth interval, number of births, sex ratio of children, and premarital pregnancy among migrants at different birth cohorts will be conducted, using data from CMDS 2015. The findings will provide evidence for the formulation and implementation of policies on marriage and childbirth among Chinese internal migrants.

2 Data and Methods

2.1 Data Source

The data were from the China Migrants Dynamic Survey (CMDS) in 2015. CMDS is a large-scale nationwide sampling survey organized by the National Health Commission of China. CMDS 2015 used the data in 2014 as the basic sampling frame, and a stratified, multi-stage and probability proportionate to size (PPS) sampling method was applied (National Health Commission of China, 2018). The detailed sampling process was reported elsewhere (Chen et al., 2017). The investigators were required to receive formal training before conducting a face-to-face interview at participants' house.

2.2 Study Participants

The participants of this survey were defined as residents aged 15 years or above (born in or before May, 2000) who had lived in local areas for at least one month before the survey but had no local *hukou*. Individuals who migrated for the purpose of study/training, tourism or medical care, individuals whose family members have local *hukou*, and soldiers were excluded. A total of 206,000 internal migrants were surveyed in CMDS 2015, and 201,310 respondents aged 15–59 years old were included in this study.

2.3 Measures

Maiden migration was defined as being away from the place of household registration for the first time and at least one month, excluding those leaving for tourism, medical treatment, business trip, or family visit (within one month). Departure from the place of household registration was evaluated based on the geographical county/district boundary, which did not include intra-county migration.

Marital status referred to the legal marital status of the respondents, which was classified into unmarried, maiden married, remarried, divorced and widowed groups. It should be noted that unmarried cohabitation was defined as being married if having pregnancy or birth. The time of first marriage was determined by the time of getting the marriage certificate. For unmarried cohabitation, the time of first marriage was the time of beginning the cohabitation.

Childbirth status referred to the status of biological children of the respondents, including children who had died or was in custody by ex-spouse after divorce, but not including children brought by current spouse of remarriage or children who were adopted. First birth interval referred to the interval between first marriage and first birth. In this study, we mainly analyzed the first birth interval of migrants in first marriage, not including the migrants whose marital status were remarriage, divorse or widow.

Intermarriage circle was measured according to the question whether the *hukou* of husband and wife were in the same province. It was considered as inter-provincial marriage when the couple's *hukou* belonged to different provinces, otherwise it was considered as inner-provincial marriage.

Premarital pregnancy consisted of two types. The first was premarital birth, it meant that the time of first marriage was later than the time of first birth. The second was shotgun marriage, the date of first marriage was earlier than the date of first birth, but the interval time was less than 9 months.

This study divided the respondents into four birth cohorts according to their experiences at the age of 14, which considered not only physiological age but also social backgrounds (Pan, White, Wang, & Laumann, 2004). The 1955–1964 cohort were influenced by the Cultural Revolution when they were 14 years old during 1969-1978. The 1965–1974 cohort experienced the early stage of the Reform and Opening Up at the age of 14 during 1979–1988. The 1975–1987 cohort entered the age of 14 during 1989–2001, the initial establishment of a market economy. The 1988–2000 cohort were exactly 14 years old in 2002–2014 when China was in the period of improving the Reform and Opening Up.

2.4 Statistical Analysis

Descriptive analysis, univariate analysis, multilevel model and Cox regression analysis were used in this study. $p < 0.05$ indicated that the difference was statistically significant. The statistical analysis was conducted by SPSS version 20.0 and SAS version 9.4.

Continuous data, such as age of first marriage, age of first childbirth, and first birth interval, were described using Median (IQR), and non-parametric test was used for bivariate analysis. Count data were described using relative numbers like proportion, and χ^2 test was used for bivariate analysis.

The multilevel model was performed to analyze the relationship between birth cohort and some marriage and childbirth outcomes, including the order between first marriage and migration, intermarriage circles, number of children, premarital pregnancy status, age of first marriage, and age of first childbearing. In the multilevel model, province was set as the macro level (level 2), and migrant was set as the individual level (level 1). Intra-class correlation coefficient (ICC) was obtained in each model.

The Cox proportional hazards regression model (forward stepwise of likelihood ratio with entry criterion of 0.05 and retention criterion of 0.10) was used to analyze the relationship between birth cohort and first birth interval. Migrants that had premarital birth were excluded in this analysis. The birth of first child was considered as survival event, the interval between marriage and the birth of first child was treated as survival time. The subjects who were childless at the time of survey were treated as censorship, and the time between first marriage and the survey was treated as censored time. In this model, a negative coefficient ($\beta_i < 0$, $RR < 1$) means a lower probability to have the first child, which implies a longer first birth interval. In contrast, a positive coefficient ($\beta_i > 0$, $RR > 1$) is an implication of a shorter first birth interval.

Because some marriage and childbirth behaviors were associated with both wives and husbands, related models were adjusted by adding the characteristics of the migrant spouse as covariates besides the respondents' characteristics.

3 Results

3.1 Characteristics of Participants

The average age of the respondents was 33 (26–41) years old. They were mainly born in 1975–87 (43.32%), followed by 1988–2000 (27.52%) and 1965–74 (23.22%). Those who born in 1955–64 accounted for only 5.95% of the total sample. Males and females accounted for about half of the total, respectively. Most of the participants graduated from junior high school (50.97%), followed by senior high school (21.96%). Only 14.36% of them received primary or less education, and 12.71% of them graduated from college or above. Han nationality was the main ethnicity of internal migrants (92.17%), and agricultural *hukou* was the main *hukou* type (84.14%). Most internal migrants migrated across provinces (50.07%), followed by cross-city within province (30.32%), and cross-county within city (19.61%). The detailed sociodemographic characteristics of migrants are shown in Table 1. In Table 1, in 1955–64 birth cohort, the proportion of male migrants accounted for 63.26%, but it decreased to 43.10% in 1988–2000 birth cohort. The educational level increased gradually from older to more recent birth cohorts.

Table 1 Socio-demographic characteristics of internal migrants at different birth cohorts [n (%)]

Variables	1955–64	1965–74	1975–87	1988–2000	Total
Gender					
Male	7572(63.26)	27,448(58.73)	47,567(54.54)	23,877(43.10)	106,464(52.89)
Female	4398(36.74)	19,288(41.27)	39,642(45.46)	31,518(56.90)	94,846(47.11)
Education					
Illiteracy	783(6.54)	1451(3.10)	794(0.91)	245(0.44)	3273(1.63)
Primary school	3581(29.92)	11,600(24.82)	8100(9.29)	2344(4.23)	2,5625(12.73)
Junior high school	5237(43.75)	25,881(55.38)	45,569(52.25)	25,918(46.79)	102,605(50.97)
Senior high school	1977(16.52)	6060(12.97)	19,268(22.09)	16,907(30.52)	44,212(21.96)
College	278(2.32)	1191(2.55)	8087(9.27)	6920(12.49)	16,476(8.18)
Bachelor's degree or above	114(0.95)	553(1.18)	5391(6.18)	3061(5.53)	9119(4.53)
Ethnicity					
Han nationality	11,063(92.42)	43,720(93.55)	80,443(92.24)	50,325(90.85)	185,551(92.17)
Minority	907(7.58)	3016(6.45)	6766(7.76)	5070(9.15)	15,759(7.83)
Hukou type					
Agricultural	9558(79.85)	40,055(85.70)	71,674(82.19)	48,102(86.83)	169,389(84.14)
Non-agricultural	2412(20.15)	6681(14.30)	15,535(17.81)	7293(13.17)	31,921(15.86)
Migration range					
Inter-provincial	5802(48.47)	24,422(52.26)	43,217(49.56)	27,362(49.39)	100,803(50.07)
Cross-city within province	3587(29.97)	13,230(28.31)	26,853(30.79)	17,367(31.35)	61,037(30.32)
Cross-county within city	2581(21.56)	9084(19.44)	17,139(19.65)	10,666(19.25)	39,470(19.61)
Total	11,970(5.95)	46,736(23.22)	87,209(43.32)	55,395(27.52)	201,310(100.00)

3.2 *Marital Status of Migrants*

3.2.1 Marital Status

First marriage was the main marital characteristic of internal migrants (77.37%), followed by unmarried (18.92%). The marital status from unmarried to married intersected 23 years old (Fig. 1).

The proportions of unmarried female migrants in all age groups were smaller than those of male migrants (Fig. 2). Started from 15 years old, the difference in unmarried proportion between male and female migrants had risen gradually, and the difference was the largest at the age of 22 (27.02%). The difference has gradually narrowed after 22 years old. In addition, as shown in Fig. 2, there were early marriages for both male and female migrants (married before 22 years for males and before 20 years for females in China), and the proportion was higher in female migrants (7.07%) (4.44% in male migrants).

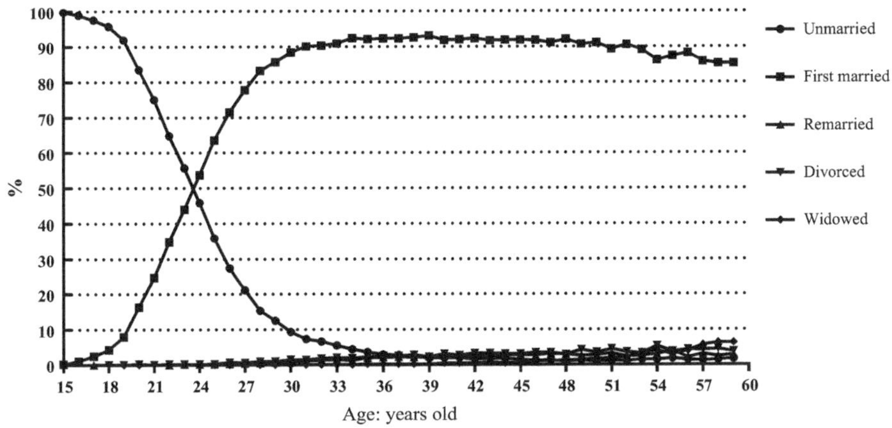

Fig. 1 Marital status of Chinese internal migrants by age, CMDS 2015

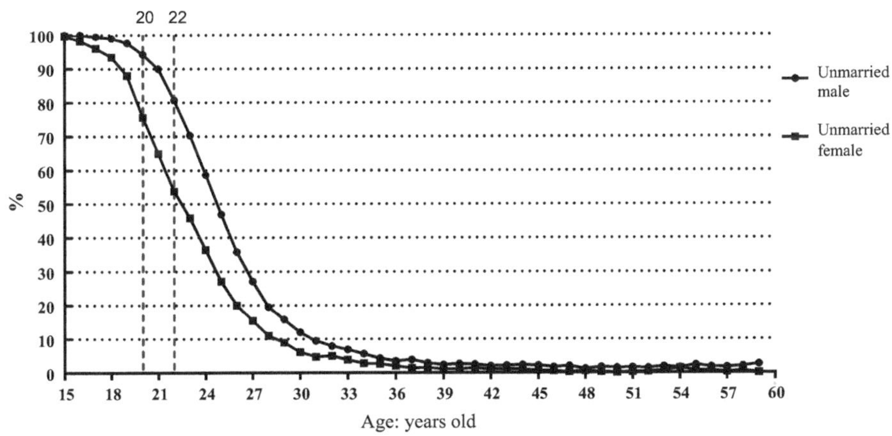

Fig. 2 Unmarried status of Chinese internal migrants by sex and age, CMDS 2015

3.2.2 First Marriage and First Migration

According to the order between first migration and first marriage, married migrants were divided into three groups: migrating after the first marriage (55.12%), migrating before the first marriage (37.60%), and migrating and getting married at the same year (7.28%). The order between first marriage and first migration at different birth cohorts is shown in Table 2. Most internal migrants born in early years migrated after their first marriage, but more recent cohorts tended to migrate before their first marriage. Only 6.13% of the 1955–64 birth cohort migrated before their first marriage, but it rose to 62.64% in 1988–2000 birth cohort.

Table 2 Marital status of internal migrants at different birth cohorts [n (%)]

Variables	Total	1955–64	1965–74	1975–87	1988–2000	$Z/\chi2$	p
The order between first marriage and first migration						31089.103	<0.001
Migration and getting married at the same year	11,873(7.28)	177(1.50)	1721(3.74)	6426(7.95)	3549(14.44)		
Migration after first marriage	89,960(55.12)	10,915(92.37)	36,534(79.40)	36,874(45.64)	5637(22.93)		
Migration before first marriage	61,369(37.60)	724(6.13)	7756(16.86)	37,488(46.40)	15,399(62.64)		
Age of the first marriage						10182.269	<0.001
M (IQR)	23(21–25)	23(21–25)	23(21–25)	23(22–26)	21(20–23)		
Intermarriage circle						1357.027	<0.001
Inter-provincial marriage	6857(4.32)	202(1.85)	851(1.93)	4073(5.15)	1731(7.09)		
Inner-provincial marriage	151,798(95.68)	10,732(98.15)	43,327(98.07)	75,042(94.85)	22,697(92.91)		

Table 3 Multilevel model of the relationship between birth cohort and the order between first marriage and migration in Chinese internal migrants ($n = 151{,}329$)

Characteristic	Variable	*β*	*Adjusted OR*	*95%CI*
Birth cohort	1955–64		1	
	1965–74	1.162	3.195	2.835–3.600
	1975–87	2.620	13.739	12.210–15.459
	1988–2000	3.780	43. 801	38.758–49.500

Note β: coefficient, *OR*: odds ratio, *CI*: confidence intervel. Adjusted for gender, education, *hukou* type, and ethnicity. The ICC was 0.123

In multilevel model analysis, because the number of internal migrants choosing to migrate and get married at the same year was too small, we excluded them and set "migration after first marriage" as the reference. The results in Table 3 show that, compared to the internal migrants in 1955–64 birth cohort, adjusted OR increased from 3.195 in 1965–74 birth cohort to 43.801 in 1988–2000 birth cohort, which indicated that internal migrants born later were more likely to migrate before their first marriage.

3.2.3 Age of First Marriage

The median age of first marriage in internal migrants was 23 years old (ranged from 14 to 56). Table 2 shows the age of first marriage among internal migrants at different birth cohorts. The median age of first marriage among the internal migrants born between 1955 and 1987 was 23, but it changed to 21 years old among the internal migrants born between 1988 and 2000 (Table 2).

The results of multilevel analysis in Table 4 show that, compared to the internal migrants in 1955–64 birth cohort, the coefficient decreased from −1.662 in 1965–74 birth cohort to −7.750 in 1988–2000 birth cohort.

Table 4 Multilevel model analysis of the relationship between birth cohort and age of first marriage in Chinese internal migrants ($n = 155{,}744$)

Characteristic	Variable	*β*	*SE*	*p*
Birth cohort	1955–64	Reference		
	1965–74	−1.662	0.080	<0.001
	1975–87	−3.977	0.085	<0.001
	1988–2000	−7.750	0.093	<0.001

Note β: coefficient, *SE*: standard error. Adjusted for migrants' order between first migration and first marriage, migrants and their spouse's education, *hukou* type, ethnicity, and spouse's age. The ICC was 0.027

Table 5 Multilevel model analysis of the relationship between birth cohort and intermarriage circle of migrants (n = 158,641)

Characteristic	Variable	β	*Adjusted OR*	*95%CI*
Birth cohort	1955–64		1	
	1965–74	−0.238	0.788	0.649–0.957
	1975–87	0.077	1.080	0.877–1.331
	1988–2000	0.262	1.300	1.030–1.640

Note β: coefficient, *OR*: odds ratio, *CI*: confidence interval. Adjusted for the migrants' order between first migration and first marriage, marital status, migrants and their spouse's education, hukou type, ethnicity, and spouse's age. The ICC was 0.100

3.2.4 Intermarriage Circle

Migrant couples were mainly from the same province (95.68%), and inter-provincial marriage only account for 4.32%. Intermarriage circles of migrants at different birth cohorts are shown in Table 4. The proportion of inter-provincial marriages increased in more recent birth cohorts. Only 1.85% of the 1955–64 birth cohort had an inter-provincial marriage, but this proportion rose to 7.09% in 1988–2000 birth cohort.

The results of multilevel model analysis ("inner-provincial marriage" as the reference) are shown in Table 5. Compared to the migrants in 1955–64 birth cohort, the adjusted OR was 0.788 in 1965–74 birth cohort and 1.300 in 1988–2000 birth cohort, which indicated that internal migrants in more recent birth cohorts were more likely to have an inter-provincial marriage.

3.3 *Childbirth Status of Migrants*

3.3.1 Number of Children

Married migrants had an average of 1 (interquartile, 1–2) children, ranging from 0 to 9. Among them, those who did not have any child accounted for 7.27%, those who had one or two children accounted for 52.57% and 34.89%, respectively, and those who had three or more children accounted for 5.27%. Table 6 shows the childbirth status of migrants at different birth cohorts. More recent birth cohorts had fewer children on average. The median number of children in the migrants born between 1955 and 1974 was 2, and it decreased to 1 in the migrants born between 1975 and 2000. Table 6 also shows the sex ratio. The overall sex ratio of migrants' children was 123.18. Compared with older migrants, the sex ratio of younger migrants' children was lower.

Table 7 shows the results of multilevel model analysis (using ">1 child" as the reference). Compared to the migrants in 1955–64 birth cohort, the adjusted OR was 0.875 in 1975–87 birth cohort and 2.646 in 1988–2000 birth cohort.

Table 6 Childbirth status of internal migrants at different birth cohorts [n (%)]

Variables	Total	1955–64	1965–74	1975–87	1988–2000	$Z/\chi 2$	p
Number of children						11641.585	<0.001
≤1	97,670(59.85)	4972(42.08)	21,507(46.74)	50,224(62.17)	20,967(85.28)		
>1	65,534(40.15)	6844(57.92)	24,506(53.26)	30,566(37.83)	3618(14.72)		
M (IQR)	1(1–2)	2(1–2)	2(1–2)	1(1–2)	1(1–1)		
Sex ratio						—	—
Ratio	123.18	124.47	128.04	122.45	110.96		
Age at first childbearing						13834.592	<0.001
M (IQR)	24(22–26)	24(22–26)	24(22–27)	24(22–27)	22(20–23)		
Premarital pregnancy						5506.325	<0.001
Pregnancy before marriage	41,713(27.58)	1977(17.29)	8905(19.83)	21,707(28.84)	9124(46.41)		
Pregnancy after marriage	109,540(72.42)	9457(82.71)	36,000(80.17)	53,547(71.16)	10,536(53.59)		
First birth interval (month)						5977.118	<0.001
M (IQR)	12(8–20)	15(10–24)	14(9–22)	12(8–20)	9(5–14)		

Table 7 Multilevel model analysis of the relationship between birth cohort and number of children in migrants ($n = 155{,}744$)

Characteristic	Variable	*β*	*Adjusted OR*	*95%CI*
Birth cohort	1955–64		1	
	1965–74	1.0338	0.925	0.835–1.026
	1975–87	1.2237	0.875	0.778–0.983
	1988–2000	2.5678	2.646	2.238–3.128

Note β: coefficient, *OR*: odds ratio, *CI*: confidence interval. Adjusted for the migrants' order between first migration and first marriage, migrants and their spouse's education, *hukou* type, ethnicity, and spouse's age. The ICC was 0.091

Table 8 Multilevel model analysis of the relationship between birth cohort and age of first childbearing in migrants ($n = 144{,}855$)

Characteristic	Variable	*β*	*SE*	*p*
Birth cohort	1955–64	Reference		
	1965–74	−1.612	0.079	<0.001
	1975–87	−4.054	0.086	<0.001
	1988–2000	−8.245	0.095	<0.001

Note β: coefficient, *SE*: standard error. Adjusted for the migrants' order between first migration and first marriage, migrants and their spouse's education, *hukou* type, ethnicity, and spouse's age. The ICC was 0.021

3.3.2 Age of First Childbearing

The median age of first childbearing was 24 (interquartile, 22–26) years old. The minimum age was 11 years old and the maximum age was 56 years old. The first childbearing age of migrants at different birth cohorts is shown in Table 6. The median age of first childbearing among the migrants born in 1955–1987 was 24 years old, but it declined to 22 (interquartile, 20–23) years old among the migrants born in 1988–2000.

The results of multilevel model are shown in Table 8. Compared to the migrants in 1955–64 birth cohort, the coefficient decreased from −1.612 in 1965–74 birth cohort to −8.245 in 1988–2000 birth cohort. Thus, the internal migrants in more recent cohorts were more likely to have children earlier.

3.3.3 Premarital Pregnancy

For the migrants who were once married and had at least one child already, 27.58% of them were pregnant before their marriage, in which 6.58% of them had their first child born before marriage and 20.99% had a shotgun marriage. The premarital pregnancy status of migrants at different birth cohorts is shown in Table 6. Less than

Table 9 Multilevel model analysis of the relationship between birth cohort and premarital pregnancy in migrants (n= 144,855)

Characteristic	Variable	β	*Adjusted OR*	*95%CI*
Birth cohort	1955–64		1	
	1965–74	−0.198	0.820	0.761–0.884
	1975–87	−0.139	0.870	0.798–0.950
	1988–2000	0.332	1.394	1.257–1.544

Note β: coefficient, *OR*: odds ratio, *CI*: confidence interval. Adjusted for the migrants' order between first migration and first marriage, intermarriage circle, migrants and their spouse's education, *hukou* type, ethnicity, and spouse's age. The ICC was 0.086

20% of the migrants born before 1974 had premarital pregnancy, but it increased to 28.84% in 1975–87 birth cohort and 46.41% in 1988–2000 birth cohort.

Table 9 shows the results of multilevel model analysis. Compared to the migrants in 1955–64 birth cohort, the adjusted OR first decreased in 1965–74 and 1975–87 birth cohorts, and then increased to 1.394 in 1988–2000 birth cohort. Thus, the internal migrants in more recent birth cohorts were more likely to get pregnant before their first marriage.

3.3.4 First Birth Interval

The average first birth interval of migrants was 12 (interquartile, 8–20) months. The first birth interval of migrants at different birth cohorts is shown in Table 6. First birth interval reduced gradually as migrants had a baby later. The first birth interval of the migrants born in 1955–64 was 15 (interquartile, 10–24) months, but it declined to 9 (interquartile, 5–14) months in 1988–2000 birth cohort migrants.

Table 10 shows the results of Cox proportional hazards model analysis. Compared to the migrants in 1955–64 birth cohort, the adjusted RR increased to 1.089 in 1988–2000 birth cohort, which indicated that the migrants in more recent birth cohorts had a higher probability to have a shorter first birth interval.

Table 10 Cox proportional hazards model analysis on the relationship between birth cohort and first birth interval in migrants (n = 146,197)

Birth cohort	β	*SE*	*Adjusted RR*	95% CI for *RR*
1955–64	Reference			
1965–74	−0.014	0.013	0.987	0.962–1.011
1975–87	−0.020	0.016	0.980	0.949–1.012
1988–2000	0.086	0.021	1.089	1.045–1.136

Note β: coefficient, *RR*: risk ratio, *CI*: confidence interval. Adjusted for the migrants' order between first migration and first marriage, intermarriage circle, the age of first marriage, migrants and their spouse's education, *hukou* type, ethnicity, and spouse's age

4 Discussion

The marital and childbirth status of migrants are considered to be significant globally (Creighton, Matthys, & Quaranta, 2012; Pernia, 1981; Priester & Haug, 1995; Yadava & Yadava, 1990). They have significant impacts not only on the living status and lifestyle of migrants and their families (Li, 2010), but also on economic prosperity and social harmony (Yan, 2015). A study conducted in Australia found that marriage reduced more than 10% labor participation among migrants from other countries (Evans, 1984). In China, most internal migrants come from rural areas, so they often have higher-level fertility than urban residents (Zheng & Yang, 2016). Most Chinese internal migrants are young people in reproductive period, so the reproductive status of them will have a huge impact on the overall fertility level (Ye, Peng, Huang, Liu, & Zhong, 2003). Under the influence of the One-Child Policy and traditional gender norms, Chinese internal migrants tend to have a male preference for bearing children (Li, Yi, & Zhang, 2011; Wu, Viisainen, & Hemminki, 2006). Unplanned births, especially those born later, are more difficult to access reproductive health services, so maternal risk and infant mortality increase (Chen, Xie, & Liu, 2007). With the full implementation of the Two-Child Policy, the marital and childbirth status of Chinese internal migrants may change and require more medical and other resources, such as sexual and reproductive health services, medical services, education, housing, employment resources and so on.

4.1 Marital Status of Migrants

The marital status of any particular population is closely related to age structure and marriage culture (Singh, 1986). This study found that first marriage was the main pattern of marriage in Chinese internal migrants, as most of them were the young. The age of 23 was the transition age from unmarried to first marriage, so the National Health Commission of China needs pay more attention to these migrants.

Migrant couples were mostly from the same province, and most internal migrants began to migrate after their first marriage. However, the proportion of migrants who chose to migrate before their first marriage and the scale of migrants with inter-provincial marriages increased across successive cohorts. More recent cohorts might be more open-minded than the earlier, and with the development of transportation system, they were more likely to migrate before their first marriage. Because of that, they had more chances to contact with people from other provinces, which contributed to a larger proportion of inter-provincial marriage. However, even in the most recent cohort, inner-provincial marriage was still the main choice and inter-provincial marriage only accounted for 7.09%.

4.2 Childbirth Status of Migrants

The birth sex ratio of entire population ranges 105–107, with a median of 105.9. However, a lower risk of mortality in female across the life course results in the final population sex ratio of 97.9–100.3 (Hesketh & Xing, 2006). China's birth sex ratio has fluctuated around 120 since 2000 (Jiang et al., 2014a). This study found that the birth sex ratio of married migrants was 123.18, which was far higher than the natural level and slightly higher than the average level of entire population in China. The gender imbalance will inevitably lead to the emergence of "leftover men", the postponement of first marriage for males, and the increase of marriage between older males and younger females. In addition, because most unmarried male migrants are in disadvantaged social and economic conditions, there are concerns that their lack of abilities to get married and the accompanying social marginalization will lead to more antisocial behaviors and violence, which will undermine social stability and security (Hesketh & Xing, 2006; Jiang et al. 2014a). Although the birth sex ratio of more recent cohorts (born in 1988–2000) had declined to 110.96, further observations are needed to monitor the change and its influence.

For the migrants who were once married and had at least one child, 27.58% of them were pregnant before their marriage, and this proportion was 46.41% in the migrants in 1988–2000 birth cohort. Premarital pregnancy may cause serious harms to migrant women. First, unmarried pregnancy may lead to miscarriage and other adverse consequences, which may harm the health of migrant women. Second, to undertake the responsibilities as a parent, pregnant migrants may rush into marriage without in-depth learning about their partners, which may easily lead to family conflicts and divorce. Moreover, as the family planning services in China are mainly provided for married people, unmarried pregnant women cannot benefit from these services (Qi et al., 2017). Premarital pregnancy may relate to the lack of consultation and guidance from family members on marriage, as well as the lack of knowledge on reproductive health. A lower rate of condom use may easily lead to the incidence of premarital pregnancy (Zheng et al., 2001). Therefore, it is necessary to strengthen the popularization of premarital sex education knowledge to make migrants realize the harmfulness and seriousness of unmarried pregnancy. It is also necessary to take more care of the premarital pregnant female migrants, especially the younger ones.

4.3 Age of First Marriage/Childbearing and First Birth Interval of Migrants

The age of first marriage and first childbirth, and the first birth interval are closely related to fertility (Chen, 1990). For the migrants in this study, the average age of first marriage was 23 (21–25) years old, the average age of first childbirth was 24 (22–26) years old, and their average first birth interval was 12 (8–20) months. For the migrants born later, the average age of first marriage and childbearing was earlier, and the first birth interval was shorter. On the one hand, the abolishment of the administrative approval system for the first child in 2004 removed the restrictions on first birth interval (Blayo, 1993; Song et al., 2012). On the other hand, it may be caused by the increasing proportion of unmarried pregnancy among younger migrants. A younger age of getting married and having first child indicates a higher fertility rate and faster population replacement rate (Kanjanapan, 1986), which may increase the number of total population in China. Moreover, the earlier the age of first birth is, the more it is likely to have insufficient family support for raising child (Zheng, 2000).

In conclusion, the overall marital status of Chinese internal migrants was stable, but the issue of premarital pregnancy was increasingly urgent. Compared to the migrants in earlier cohorts, the migrants in more recent cohorts (born in 1988–2000) had a higher proportion of marriage after migration and inter-provincial marriage, a younger age of first marriage and first childbearing, a shorter first birth interval, a smaller number of children, a lower birth sex ratio, and a higher proportion of premarital pregnancy.

Strengths and Limitations

The data used came from a nationally representative survey. A strict quality control was adopted in every stage of the survey. The survey involved different aspects of marriage and childbearing, so it can be used to comprehensively analyze the marital and childbearing situation of Chinese internal migrants.

There are several limitations in this study. First, when analyzing the childbirth status of migrants at different cohorts, most migrants were still in their childbearing period. The current childbirth status could not fully represent the lifelong fertility of these generations. Second, when using Cox proportional hazards model to analyze the relationship between birth cohort and first birth interval, migrants having premarital birth were excluded, so the effect of cohort might be underestimated. Third, migrants who had not legal marriage but had pregnancy or birth were not included in analysis on the status of premarital pregnancy. However, the number of this group is usually small in the context of Chinese culture, so it will not have obvious effect on the status of premarital pregnancy among migrants.

References

Addo, F. R. (2014). Debt, cohabitation, and marriage in young adulthood. *Demography, 51*(5), 1677–1701.

Allendorf, K., & Pandian, R. K. (2016). The decline of arranged marriage? Marital change and continuity in India. *Population and Development Review, 42*(3), 435–464.

Blayo, Y. (1993). Control of fertility in the People's Republic of China. *Entre Nous* (22–23), e19.

Boulier, B., & Rosenzweig, M. R. (1978). Age, biological factors, and socioeconomic determinants of fertility: A new measure of cumulative fertility for use in the empirical analysis of family size. *Demography, 15*(4), 487–497.

Cai, Y., Wang, Y., Zheng, Z., Wang, J., Yao, W., & Ma, J. (2013). Predictors of reducing sexual and reproductive risk behaviors based on the information-motivation-behavioral skills (IMB) model among unmarried rural-to-urban female migrants in Shanghai, China. *Plos One, 8*(4), e62787.

Carlson, E. D. (1985). The impact of international migration upon the timing of marriage and childbearing. *Demography, 22*(1), 61–72.
Chen, F., Liu, H., Vikram, K., & Guo, Y. (2015). For better or worse: The health implications of marriage separation due to migration in rural China. *Demography, 52*(4), 1321–1343.
Chen, J., Xie, Z., & Liu, H. (2007). Son preference, use of maternal health care, and infant mortality in rural China, 1989–2000. *Population Studies, 61*(2), 161–183.
Chen, P. (1990). Changes in fertility in rural China: A simulated micro-analysis of the interactions between the demand and supply of children, and the family planning policy. *Chinese Journal of Population Science, 2*(3), 207–218.
Chen, W., Zhang, Q., Renzaho, A., Zhou, F., Zhang, H., & Ling, L. (2017). Social health insurance coverage and financial protection among rural-to-urban internal migrants in China: Evidence from a nationally representative cross-sectional study. *BMJ Global Health, 2*(4), e000477.
Creighton, M. J., Matthys, C., & Quaranta, L. (2012). Migrants and the diffusion of low marital fertility in Belgium. *Journal of Interdisciplinary History, 42*(4), 593–614.
Evans, M. D. R. (1984). Immigrant women in Australia: Resources, family and work. *International Migration Review, 18*(s4), 1063–1090.
Goodkind, D. (2017). The astonishing population averted by China's birth restrictions: Estimates, nightmares, and reprogrammed ambitions. *Demography, 54*(4), 1375–1400.
He, D., Zhou, Y., Ji, N., Wu, S., Wang, Z., Decat, P., et al. (2012). Study on sexual and reproductive health behaviors of unmarried female migrants in China. *Journal of Obstetrics and Gynaecology Research, 38*(4), 632–638.
Hesketh, T., & Xing, Z. (2006). Abnormal sex ratios in human populations: Causes and consequences. *Proceedings of the National Academy of Sciences of the United States of America, 103*(36), 13271–13275.
Islam, N. M., & Ahmed, A. U. (1998). Age at first marriage and its determinants in Bangladesh. *Asia-Pacific Population Journal, 13*(2), 73–92.
Jiang, Q., Feldman, M. W., & Li, S. (2014a). Marriage squeeze, never-married proportion, and mean age at first marriage in China. *Population Research and Policy Review, 33*(2), 189–204.
Jiang, Q., Li, Y., & Sánchez-Barricarte, J. J. (2014b). The risk of mothers' losing an only child in China. *Journal of Biosocial Science, 46*(4), 531–545.
Kanjanapan, W. (1986). Age at first marital union and fertility: Evidence from some Asian and Pacific countries. *Journal of Population Studies* (9), 79–104.
Li, H., Yi, J., & Zhang, J. (2011). Estimating the effect of the one-child policy on the sex ratio imbalance in China: Identification based on the difference-in-differences. *Demography, 48*(4), 1537–1557.
Li, R. (2010). Chances and costs: The changes in the young female's employment, education and marital status in China's metropolis. *South China Population, 25*(2), 25–31.
Liu, Z., Zhu, M., Dib, H., Li, Z., Shi, S., & Wang, Z. (2011). RH knowledge and service utilization among unmarried rural-to-urban migrants in three major cities, China. *BMC Public Health, 11*(1), e74.
Manglos-Weber, N. D., & Weinreb, A. (2017). Own-choice marriage and fertility in Turkey. *Journal of Marriage and Family, 79*(2), 372–389.
Nath, D. C., Singh, K. K., Land, K. C., & Talukdar, P. K. (1993). Age of marriage and length of the first birth interval in a traditional Indian society: Life table and hazards model analysis. *Human Biology, 65*(5), 783–797.
National Bureau of Statistics (2018). *China statistical yearbook 2017*. Beijing: China Statistics Press.
Nenko, I., & Jasienska, G. (2013). First birth interval, an indicator of energetic status, is a predictor of lifetime reproductive strategy. *American Journal of Human Biology, 25*(1), 78–82.
Nguyen, L., Nguyen, M. T., Swenson, I., & Pham, B. S. (1993). Selected determinants of fertility in Vietnam: Age at marriage, marriage to first birth interval and age at first birth. *Journal of Biosocial Science, 25*(3), 303–310.

National Health Commission of China. (2018). Introduction of migrants population dynamic monitoring survey data. Retrieved from http://www.chinaldrk.org.cn/wjw/.

Pan, S., White, W., Wang, A., & Laumann. (2004). *Sexual behavior and relation in contemporary China*. Beijing: China Social Science Documentation Publishing House.

Patravali, P., & Gaonkar, V. (1991). Opinions of educated youth towards age at marriage and difference in age between partners. *Indian Journal of Behaviour, 15*(2), 35–39.

Pernia, E. (1981). On the relationship between migration and fertility. *The Philippine Review of Economics & Business, 18*(3–4), 192–202.

Priester, T., & Haug, W. (1995). Migration and marital status. The case of Switzerland. *Schweizerische Zeitschrift für Volkswirtschaft und Statistik, 131*(2), 179–202.

Qi, J., & Yang, H. (2015). Enlargement of the marital circle, gender and premarital pregnancy in migrants families. *South China Population, 30*(4), 1–11.

Qi, S., Bao, H., Zhang, M., Yu, Y., & Liu, X. (2017). An analysis on marriage and fertility status among migrant married women of childbearing age in Jilin province. *Population Journal, 39*(1), 50–57.

Rosenwalke, I. (1972). Factors associated with religious and civil marriages. *Demography, 9*(1), 129–141.

Rundquist, F.-M., & Brown, L. A. (1989). Migrant fertility differentials in Ecuador. *Geografiska Annaler Series B Human Geography, 71b*(2), 109–123.

Shayan, Z., Ayatollahi, S. M., Zare, N., & Moradi, F. (2014). Prognostic factors of first birth interval using the parametric survival models. *International Journal of Reproductive BioMedicine, 12*(2), 125–130.

Singh, J. P. (1986). Marital status differentials in rural to city migration in India. *Genus, 42*(3–4), 89–106.

Song, Y., Zhang, L., & Duan, C. (2012). Tradition, shock and transformation: The characteristics of young migrants' marital and child-bearing behavior. *Population & Economics* (6), 8–15.

Wang, L. (2013). A study on the change of geographical marriage circle in rural China and its causes. *China Rural Survey* (5), 70–77.

Wang, Y., Yao, W., Shang, M., Cai, Y., Shi, R., Ma, J., et al. (2013). Sexual and reproductive health among unmarried rural-urban female migrants in Shanghai China: A comparative analysis. *International Journal of Environmental Research and Public Health, 10*(8), 3578–3589.

Webster, A., & Mawer, G. E. (1989). Seizure frequency and major life events in epilepsy. *Epilepsia, 30*(2), 162–167.

Wu, Z., Viisainen, K., & Hemminki, E. (2006). Determinants of high sex ratio among newborns: A cohort study from rural Anhui province, China. *Reproductive Health Matters, 14*(27), 172–180.

Yadava, K. N., & Yadava, G. S. (1990). Socioeconomic factors and effect on fertility of husband-wife separation due to migration. *Biology and Society: The Journal of the Eugenics Society, 7*(3), 139–144.

Yan, Z. (2015). Changes characteristics of the marriage status of the floating population in Guangdong. *Northwest Population Journal, 36*(4), 114–117.

Ye, J., Peng, Q., Huang, C., Liu, J., & Zhong, Z. (2003). Floating population in Guangdong. *South China Population, 18*(1), 54–64.

Zheng, Z. (2000). Social-demographic influence on first birth interval in China, 1980–1992. *Journal of Biosocial Science, 32*(3), 315–327.

Zheng, Z. (2013). The changes of temporary migrants in China and policy implication. *Chinese Journal of Population Science* (1), 36–45.

Zheng, Z., & Yang, G. (2016). Internal migration in China: Changes and trends *contemporary demographic transformations in China, India and Indonesia* (pp. 223–237). Springer.

Zheng, Z., Zhou, Y., Zheng, L., Yang, Y., Zhao, D., Lou, C., et al. (2001). Sexual behaviour and contraceptive use among unmarried, young women migrant workers in five cities in China. *Reproductive Health Matters, 9*(17), 118–127.

Zhu, N. (2002). The impacts of income gaps on migration decisions in China. *China Economic Review, 13*(2–3), 213–230.

Chapter 9
Age at Marriage and First Birth Interval Among Female Internal Migrants

Tiantian He

1 Introduction

Women's first marriage age and first birth interval are of great significance for population reproduction, which directly affect the reproductive cycle, time interval, and speed of population growth. They are also important indicators to describe female marital status and their level of fertility (Guo, 2003). Meanwhile, birth interval also reflects women's social status and gender role (Nath, Land, & Goswami, 1999).

Since the 1970s, China's family planning policy has changed from advocating 'Wan, Xi, Shao' to strictly enforcing the One-Child Policy, and to the opening up of the Two-Child Policy until now. Social factors, such as the urbanization, advancement of women's status, as well as the change of demographic factors including age structure of fertile women and marital status, have a profound effect on the reproductive behaviour of women in China. In the 1970s, the average age at marriage of women increased rapidly by 2.83 years, while the first birth interval reduced by 1.1 years (Cai, 1991). By the 1980s, age at marriage fell and the first birth interval further reduced (Zeng, 1992). However, some opposite phenomena appeared in the 1990s. The average marriage age showed an upward tendency (Lu & Wang, 2013) and the first birth interval showed an enlarging trend in fluctuation (Guo, 2003). In the 21st century, women's age at first marriage has still been slowly growing (Fu, Zhang, & Li 2013). Prior studies have shown that the age of women registered for marriage in Beijing increased by 1 year from 2004 to 2011 and female migrants in Beijing also raised their marriage age (Gao & Wu, 2012). In addition, the first birth interval also increased by 0.11–0.27 year in the 2000s (Fu, Wang, & Zeng, 2012).

As a unique group, the number of internal migrants has rapidly increased accompanied by the urbanization of China. Most internal migrants are young adults aged 18–45 years, containing great fertility potentialities (Jin, Peng, Li, Guo, & Yang,

T. He (✉)
School of Health Sciences, Wuhan University, Wuhan, China
e-mail: htt2011@whu.edu.cn

P. Wang (ed.), *The Health Status of Internal Migrants in China*,
https://doi.org/10.1007/978-981-15-4415-6_9

2005). Therefore, the fertility level of them has attracted extensive attention of family planning authorities and the community (Li & Guo, 2014). More and more females going out as migrant workers have subverted conventional gender roles and the division of labour (Silvey & Elmhirst, 2003). Besides, the culture shift caused by their migration from rural to urban areas has also changed their attitudes and behaviours towards marriage and childbearing. Prior evidence has shown that migrants' fertility rate was lower than that of rural residents, but slightly higher than that of urban dwellers (Chen, 2005; Chen & Wu, 2006; Guo, 2010). Migrating before marriage and experiences of working out of home obviously delay the age of female marriage (Liu, 2014; Xu, 2015) and shorten their first birth interval (Wu, Li, & Yue, 2006). Factors that influence their first birth interval are multiple and complicated, because fertility is not only a physiological phenomenon, but also a social phenomenon. Thus, in female's reproductive age, individual and contextual factors may both affect their birth interval (Guo & Li, 2006). Women's individual characteristics, including education, age at marriage, marriage cohort, breastfeeding time and menstrual status, have been confirmed to relate to their first birth interval (Begna, Assegid, Kassahun, & Gerbaba, 2013; Löfstedt, Ghilagaber, Shusheng, & Johansson, 2005; Sedigheh & Piri, 2012; Singh, Tripathi, Kalaivani, Singh, & Dwivedi, 2012; Shayan, Ayatollahi, Zare, & Moradi, 2014). Also, the first birth interval of urban women is longer than that of rural women (Li & Jiang, 2009; Zheng, 1999). Social contexts such as war environment and great recession may also influence female's first birth interval. Socioeconomic status (SES) determines the nutritional level of women, while the first birth interval can be used as an indicator of nutrient supply (Jampaklay, 2006; Nenko, Hayward, & Lummaa, 2014). Thus, there is also a correlation between SES and the first birth interval of females. Due to the hardness of regulation to migrants, it is difficult to collect large samples of female migrants' reproductive history data, so there are few researches on the first birth interval among internal migrants in China. Liang (2016) studied the influencing factors of each birth interval among internal migrants in Shanghai, China, and found that their age and education were significantly related to their birth interval. Chen and Ye (2009) found that individual characteristics, migration experiences, family relationships and social networks all affected the first birth interval of internal migrants in Xiamen, China. The number of Chinese internal migrants reached 247 million in 2015 and was expected to grow at the speed of 6–7 million people per year before 2020 (National Health Commission of China, 2016). The change in the pattern of marriage and fertility among migrants may also have a profound impact on China's population development. Therefore, the purpose of this chapter was to examine the change in age at marriage and first birth interval, and to explore the influencing factors of first birth interval among Chinese internal migrants using nationally representative data collected in 2014.

2 Data and Methods

2.1 Data Source

The data used for this study were from the China Migrants Dynamic Survey (CMDS) in 2014, and the respondents investigated covered all 31 provinces in mainland China. In this survey, respondents are internal migrants aged 15–59 years who have lived in current city for at least one month, excluding migrants surveyed in station, dock, airport, hotels and hospitals. A stratified, multi-stage sampling and probability-proportional-to-size sampling (PPS) sampling method was used.

This survey collects demographic data and complete reproductive history of female migrants, and this study selected 67,714 married women as valid samples from 200,937 valid questionnaires. To facilitate the analysis of trends on first marriage age and first birth interval in different time periods, the sample used was divided into nine marriage cohorts: 1969–1975, 1976–1980, 1981–1985, 1986–1990, 1991–1995, 1996–2000, 2001–2005, 2006–2010, and 2011–2014 according to the year of marriage. The first birth interval refers to the time between marriage and first birth (or expiration date of the survey), which is measured in month. It is noted that some married women (n = 16,708) are pregnant or give birth before marriage, so the first birth interval of them is within eight months or less than zero. In the survival analysis, cases whose first birth interval is negative are automatically removed. Some women (n = 4,593) do not have children before the survey and they are considered as censored cases in survival analysis. For these samples, the first birth interval of censored cases meant the time between marriage and survey.

2.2 Statistical Methods

Fertility events consist of two outcomes, including fertility time (continuous variable) and having children or not (dichotomous variable). Censored cases would be lost and a biased estimate might be yielded if using ordinary least squares (OLS) or binary logistic regression analysis. Thus, survival analysis is adopted in this study to analyse the first birth interval of migrant females. Survival curves of first birth interval are drawn using Kaplan-Meier method. Most women choose to have their first child within five years after marriage, and Breslow test is more sensitive to early disparity in observation. Therefore, Breslow test is chosen to compare first birth interval disparities in different subgroups. The COX proportional hazard model, a kind of semiparametric model, is used to compare the risk of first birth, and a shorter first birth interval means a greater risk of first birth. In this model, female's first birth interval and birth status are used as dependent variables; women's sociodemographic characteristics, including ethnicity, education, *hukou*, migration experience, range of migration, family income, willingness of long-term residence, age at marriage and marriage cohort, are used as independent variables.

3 Results

3.1 Basic Information

Table 1 shows the basic information of the sample used, and a Kaplan-Meier method is used to examine the differences in first birth interval between or among subgroups. The results show that 93.1% of the respondents are Han nationality, over 70.0% of them have an education of middle (junior or senior high) school or above, and 84.3% of them are from rural areas. In addition, most of the respondents are pregnant before migration, and over 60.0% of them have a willingness of long-term residence in local areas.

The average first birth interval in Table 1 is not an arithmetic mean commonly used, but an approximate mean estimated by specific method in survival analysis because of the existence of censored cases. The results of Breslow tests show that the mean value of first birth interval among females with different ethnicity, education, *hukou*, family income, willingness of long-term residence, migration experience and marriage cohort are statistically significant. For *hukou*, other types of *hukou*, including residents *hukou* transformed by agricultural or non-agricultural *hukou*, are excluded.

3.2 Age at First Marriage and First Birth Interval

Table 2 and Fig. 1 show the age at first marriage and age at first birth of female migrants. The marriage age and age at first birth both show a tendency of increase, and the first marriage age rises from 18.01 to 20.50 across the successive cohorts. Specifically speaking, the age at first marriage and age at first birth largely increased in the first two marriage cohorts, and they gradually increased across the following successive cohorts. The age at marriage and age at first birth almost changed synchronously, and the first birth interval reduced with successive marriage cohorts, especially in more recent cohorts. That is to say, the first birth interval has undergone a subtle change with time. As can be seen in Table 1, the respondents in more recent marriage cohort have a shorter first birth interval, except that the first birth interval of 1996–2000 marriage cohort rises to 24.77 months. The average first birth interval significantly decreases from 45.43 months in the oldest marriage cohort to 20.63 months and 16.54 months in more recent marriage cohorts. Fig. 2 also shows that the first marriage age of the most recent marriage cohort is very close to the age at first childbearing, which can be ascribed to two reasons. One is the selection bias of the samples, as female migrants that tend to procreate earlier are covered in this cohort due to the short interval between investigation and marriage. The other is that a large number of premarital pregnancy cases existed in this marriage cohort reduce the age at first birth.

Table 1 Basic information of 67,714 married women aged 15–59 in China

Variables	n	Percent (%)	First Birth interval		*p*
			Mean	SE	
Ethnicity					<0.001
Han nationality	59681	93.13	27.56	0.31	
Minority	4401	6.87	31.23	1.18	
Education					<0.001
Primary school or below	12439	19.41	25.73	0.52	
Junior high school	34262	53.47	25.96	0.37	
Senior high school	10876	16.97	29.86	0.79	
College or above	6505	10.15	37.78	1.41	
Hukou					<0.001
Agricultural	53997	84.26	25.55	0.29	
Non-agricultural	9321	14.55	41.49	1.19	
Others	764	1.19	29.31	2.44	
Family income monthly (CNY)					<0.001
<= 2500	5507	8.59	42.88	1.45	
2501–5000	29234	45.62	28.06	0.44	
5001–10000	25196	39.32	23.08	0.32	
>10000	4144	6.47	25.76	0.94	
Range of migration					0.086
Inter-provincial	32536	50.77	28.02	0.42	
Corss-city within province	19314	30.14	27.62	0.51	
Cross-county within city	12232	19.09	26.37	0.60	
Willingness of long-term residence					0.005
Yes	39549	61.72	25.21	0.31	
No	7119	11.11	31.01	1.01	
Not clear	17413	27.17	32.88	0.72	
Migration before pregnancy					<0.001
Yes	17587	29.56	19.04	0.16	
No	41902	70.44	18.07	0.09	
Marriage cohort					<0.001
1969–1975	97	0.15	45.43	9.63	
1976–1980	827	1.29	45.44	3.08	
1981–1985	2597	4.05	30.46	1.17	
1986–1990	6420	10.02	26.79	0.61	
1991–1995	8424	13.15	23.22	0.40	

(continued)

Table 1 (continued)

Variables	n	Percent (%)	First Birth interval		p
			Mean	SE	
1996–2000	10475	16.35	24.77	0.34	
2001–2005	11720	18.29	21.52	0.24	
2006–2010	14882	23.22	20.63	0.19	
2011–2014	8640	13.48	16.54	0.15	

Note SE: standard error, CNY: Chinese Yuan

Table 2 First marriage age and first birth age in different marriage cohorts

Marriage cohort	First marriage age			First Birth age		
	Mean	95% confidence interval		Mean	95% confidence interval	
		Lower	Upper		Lower	Upper
1969–1975	18.01	17.70	18.32	19.99	19.39	20.60
1976–1980	20.86	20.70	21.02	23.11	22.86	23.35
1981–1985	20.86	20.77	20.95	22.61	22.49	22.72
1986–1990	21.14	21.08	21.19	22.75	22.67	22.82
1991–1995	21.83	21.78	21.88	23.31	23.24	23.37
1996–2000	22.66	22.60	22.71	24.15	24.09	24.22
2001–2005	22.91	22.85	22.96	24.22	24.16	24.28
2006–2010	23.42	23.37	23.48	24.34	24.28	24.40
2011–2014	24.50	24.43	24.57	24.62	24.53	24.70

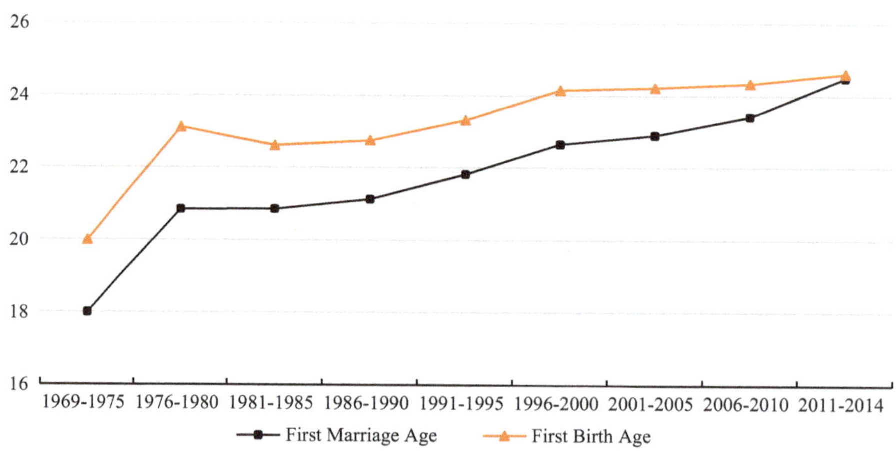

Fig. 1 First marriage age and first birth age in different marriage cohorts

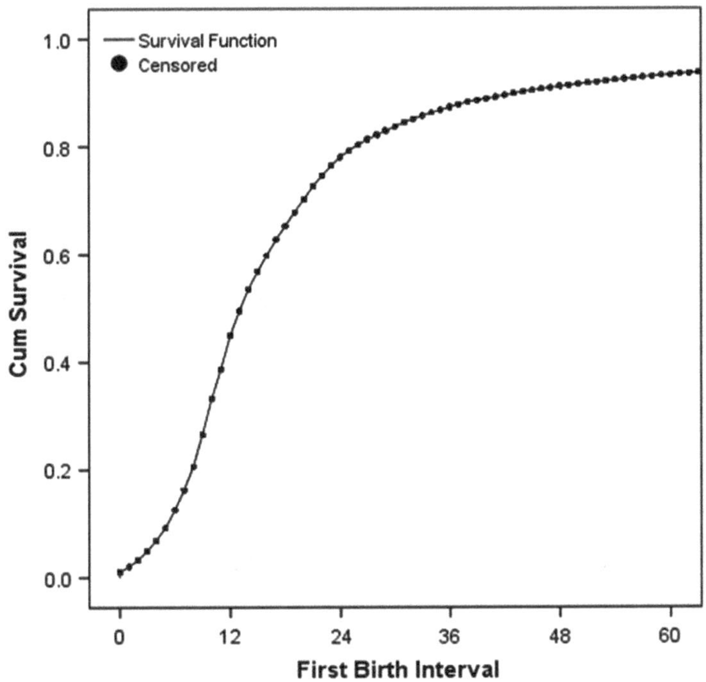

Fig. 2 Survival function of first birth interval

Figure 2 depicts the survival curve of first birth interval in five years including censored cases, plotted by the first birth interval on the horizontal axis measured in months and the probability of first birth on the vertical axis. The curve shows that nearly half women choose to have their first child within one year after marriage, 80% women choose to have their first child within two years after marriage, almost 90% women choose to have their first child within three years after marriage, and only a few of them have a baby after three years of marriage.

To show the distribution of first birth interval across successive marriage cohorts more clearly, the survival curves of nine marriage cohorts are illustrated in Fig. 3. Graphs within three years after marriage are shown, because almost 90% women have completed childbearing in this period. The curves hardly overlap within two years after marriage, indicating there are significant differences among marriage cohorts during this period. These curves tend to be higher in more recent marriage cohorts, indicating that more recent marriage cohorts tend to have a shorter first birth interval. The curve of marriage cohorts after 1980 begin to coincide when the childbearing is completed after two years of marriage, indicating that there is no significant difference among marriage cohorts in this period.

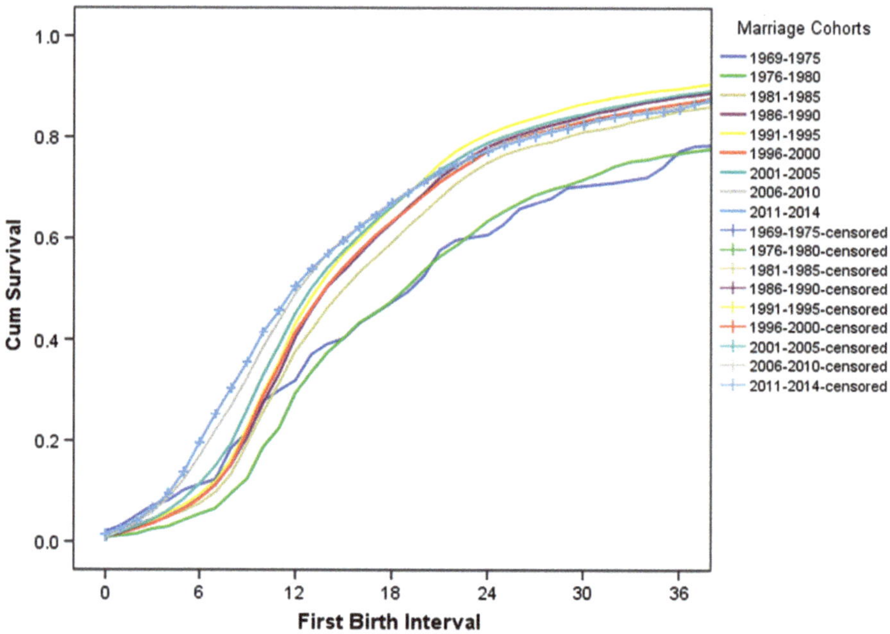

Fig. 3 Survival function of first birth interval in different marriage cohorts

3.3 *Influencing Factors of First Birth Interval*

In the COX proportional hazard model, forward method is used to select each variable in turn. Income is included in the model in the form of logarithm due to its skewed distribution. The inclusion criteria is $p < 0.05$ and the exclusion criteria is $p > 0.1$. The final model is shown in Table 3.

The results in Table 3 show that the first birth risk of minorities is 14% lower than that of the Han nationality, indicating that minorities have a longer first birth interval ($p < 0.001$). Females with more education have a longer first birth interval. Compared with women with primary school education or below, the first birth risk is 10.4% ($p < 0.001$) lower among women with senior high school education and 31.6% ($p < 0.001$) lower among women with college education or above. The first birth risk for females with non-agricultural *hukou* is 13.8% ($p < 0.001$) lower than that with agricultural *hukou*, illustrating that females with non-agricultural *hukou* have a longer first birth interval. The first birth risk of females who have migration experiences before pregnancy is 16.7% ($p < 0.001$) lower than that with no migration experience before pregnancy, so females who have migrated before pregnancy have a longer first birth interval. The risk of first birth increases by 12.9% ($p < 0.001$) with every additional unit of family monthly income, indicating that females with more family income have a shorter first birth interval. A gradual increase of firth birth risk

Table 3 Influencing factors of first birth interval: based on the Cox model

Variables	b	SE	Wald	*p*	HR
Ethnicity (ref: Han nationality)					
Minority	−0.149	0.017	80.345	<0.001	0.861
Education (ref: Primary school or below)					
Junior high school	−0.012	0.011	1.081	0.298	0.988
Senior high school	−0.110	0.015	52.684	<0.001	0.896
College or above	−0.380	0.021	339.090	<0.001	0.684
Hukou (ref: Agricultural)					
Non-agricultural household	−0.148	0.014	119.551	<0.001	0.862
Migration before pregnancy (ref: No)					
Yes	−0.184	0.010	360.611	<0.001	0.833
Range of migration (ref: Inter-provincial)					
Corss-city within province	0.031	0.010	10.284	0.001	1.031
Cross-county within city	0.030	0.011	6.939	0.008	1.030
Family income monthly (CNY)	0.121	0.018	45.310	<0.001	1.129
Marriage cohort (ref: 1969–1975)					
1976–1980	−0.022	0.113	0.037	0.848	0.979
1981–1985	0.193	0.109	3.143	0.076	1.212
1986–1990	0.272	0.108	6.413	0.011	1.313
1991–1995	0.357	0.107	11.065	0.001	1.430
1996–2000	0.333	0.107	9.590	0.002	1.395
2001–2005	0.482	0.108	20.071	<0.001	1.619
2006–2010	0.709	0.108	43.365	<0.001	2.032
2011–2014	1.276	0.108	138.707	<0.001	3.583
First marriage age	−0.007	0.001	26.038	<0.001	0.993

Note b means coefficient, SE means standard error, HR means hazard ratio

across successive marriage cohorts is also observed. The first birth risk of 1991–1995 marriage cohort is 43.0% higher than that of the reference group (1969–1975 marriage cohort), the first birth risk of 2006–2010 marriage cohort is about twice as much as the reference group, and the first birth risk of the most recent marriage cohort is more than three times greater than the reference group. Thus, a more recent marriage cohort usually have a shorter first birth interval.

4 Discussion

4.1 Rise of Age at First Marriage and Decline of First Birth Interval

First marriage age shows a tendency of increase. The average age at marriage is 18.01 years old in 1969–1975 marriage cohort, and it rises to 24.50 in 2011–2014 marriage cohort. These results are consistent with some previous studies. Cai (1991) found a steady rise of the first marriage age from 1949 to 1979, with a rapid growth in 1970s, in Chinese females; however, the marriage age began to decline in the early 1980s, remained stable for the next three years and significantly rose after 1987. Wang and Yang (1996) also found that the first marriage age has increased rapidly in the 1970s and decreased in the early 1980s. Guo (2003) studied the age at first marriage of Chinese women in 1990s and found a continuous increase of the average age at first marriage since the 1990s.

China's family planning policy is considered the most important factor that leads to the rapid increase of first marriage age among Chinese women in the 1970s. As a basic requirement for population control, the family planning policy of 'Wan, Xi, Shao' was put forward in the 1960s and had formally implemented nationwide since 1971. 'Wan' meant later marriage, and brides over 23 and grooms over 25 were commonly considered later marriage, which was officially encouraged. However, the legal marriage age for women was 18 years old in that era. It was the policies requirement that led to a significant increase in women's marriage age. In the early 1980s, the first marriage age ceased to rise, mainly because the 'One-Child Policy' was enacted in 1979, and the new marital law set women's legal marriage age as 20 years old. Thus, a 'wedding hot' appeared in that period. Due to the difficulty of the family planning policy implementation among internal migrants (mainly rural-to-urban migrants that migrate from rural to urban China), the age at first marriage in the 1970s did not evidently rise. In Table 3.2, the first marriage age in the early 1980s is 20.86 years, which is significantly lower than the policy requirement (23 years old) and findings from other studies (22 years old). Therefore, the first marriage age in the early 1980s did not decline, which is not in line with the results from some previous studies (Wang & Yang, 1996). For 1986 to 2014 marriage cohorts, the average age at first marriage has increased steadily and slowly across successive cohorts, which can mainly attribute to multiple social factors. Prior studies have found that the social environment of gender roles (Ono, 2003), and women's employment status (Oppenheimer, 1988), education (Shafer & Qian, 2010) and migration experience (Jampaklay, 2006) all have an impact on women's first marriage age. During 1986 to 2014, with the rapid development of social economy and increasing open environment in China, women's social status has greatly improved, as they can receive more education and have more job opportunities. Females put more emphasize on their independence and do not regard marriage as the only prospect. Arranged marriage reduces, free love and free marriage are esteemed, and women have more freedom to choose marriage partner, looking for a soul mate, and no longer take birth as the only purpose of marriage. In addition, receiving more education also increases their first marriage age (Wang & Yang, 1996).

By contrast, the first birth interval of female migrants has reduced gradually across successive marriage cohorts, which seems to run counter to the declining fertility rate in China. However, similar evidence can be found in some previous studies. Wang and Yang (1996) reported the first birth interval of Chinese females decreased from 34 months in the 1950s to less than 18 months in the 1980s. Similarly, a study in Yunnan Province also finds that the first birth interval of females decreased from 34 months to 12 months during 1936–1975 (Löfstedt, Ghilagaber, Shusheng, & Johansson, 2005).

The argument that the rise in the first marriage age leads to the decline in the first birth interval has also been discussed in many prior studies. The first marriage age is influenced by policies and many other social factors, while the age at first birth is only affected by the social change (Zheng, 2000). Thus, as shown in this chapter, the first birth age has a smaller increase than the age at first marriage, resulting in the decline of first birth interval.

4.2 *Influencing Factors of First Birth Interval*

As some scholars have mentioned, the influencing factors of first birth interval are complex and diverse. Prior studies have shown that the first birth interval is highly related to conscious contraceptive behaviours, which are affected by the willingness of fertility and contraceptive knowledge (Zheng, 2000). By contrast, some studies have indicated that first birth interval only reflects individual physiological status without consideration of contraception and induced abortion (Li & Jiang, 2009).

The COX proportional hazard model indicates that women' ethnicity, education, *hukou*, migration experience, family income and marriage cohorts have great impacts on their first birth interval. The first birth interval of minorities is longer than that of the Han nationality. There is a difference in the urgency to have a child between different ethnicities. It reflects why the Han nationality is growing faster than minorities from one side. Prior studies also suggest that there may be differences in the intercultural physiology that influences birth interval (Shi & Li, 2004). Second, more education relates to a longer first birth interval, which can attribute to their contraceptive behaviours. Females with more education usually have a higher socioeconomic status and their opportunity cost of childbearing is greater (Fu et al., 2013), so their willingness of fertility is not strong. Besides, they have easier access to contraceptive knowledge and contraceptive tools, so they have more opportunities to prevent pregnancy after marriage. Third, urban female migrants have a longer first birth interval than rural female migrants, which can attribute to the difference in culture environment. In rural China, females are required early fertility according to traditional customs, they suffer more stress from their families and friends. By contrast, more job opportunities for urban females improve their social status and reduce pressures from family and acquaintances. Urban females no longer regard fertility as the central task of marriage, which also increases the possibility of contraception after marriage. Fourth, females who have migrated before pregnancy have a longer first birth interval than those who have not, because their fertility behaviours are similar to urban females after they migrated from rural to urban areas. This is a testament that further verifies the importance of social environment and culture for fertility. Fifth, more family income relates to a shorter first birth interval, which may be related to the economic cost of childbearing (Chen & Ye, 2009). The family with better economic conditions has less concern for the economic cost of childbearing, so the likelihood of fertility increases. The results show that younger marriage cohort has a shorter first birth interval, which mainly relates to physiological factors. As time progresses and social culture becomes open, the attitude towards sex behaviour is increasingly tolerant. Premarital sex that is unacceptable in the old days has become widespread. Sexual behaviours have a direct impact on female's first birth interval. High-frequency sexual behaviours relate to a shorter interval required for pregnancy after marriage. In the arranged marriage in the old days, the couples were not allowed to see each other before marriage, and this kind of strangeness usually leads to low-frequency sexual behaviours after marriage. However, with the improvement of women' social status, going out for work gives females opportunities to meet a variety of people and to choose their lovers. This kind of marriage because of love can increase the frequency of sexual behaviour and the risk of pre-marital pregnancy (Rindfuss & Morgan, 1983). Although many literatures have suggested that first marriage age affects first birth interval, our results show a different result, probably because the effect of first marriage age on the first birth interval is not linear (Zheng, 2000).

5 Conclusions and Limitations

This study shows that the age at first marriage rises across successive marriage cohorts, while the first birth interval declines. The influencing factors of first birth interval are complex and diverse. Female migrants' ethnicity, education, *hukou*, migration experience, family income, marriage cohort are related to their first birth interval. It is worth noting that this chapter finds the first birth age has an increasing trend, which needs to be paid attention to by relevant personnels of maternal and child health. Because the birth age would pose a threat to the health of mothers and newborns if it exceeds the optimal childbearing age. However, limited to the research data and methods, there are some limitations in this study. First, due to the lack of data, no variable that can directly reflect female contraceptive behaviours (e.g., contraceptive method and time) is used or controlled for. Differences in contraceptive behaviours are speculated only through the social characteristics of female migrants. Second, due to the regional difference in fertility behaviour, female migrants in the same area may be homogeneous in childbearing behaviours, and the ordinal COX model may yield biased estimations. Thus, a multilevel model should be used to examine the effect of both regional and individual factors on first birth interval.

References

Begna, Z., Assegid, S., Kassahun, W., & Gerbaba, M. (2013). Determinants of inter birth interval among married women living in rural pastoral communities of southern Ethiopia: A case control study. *BMC Pregnancy and Childbirth, 13*(1), 116.

Cai, D. (1991). The change of age at first marriage, first birth of Chinese females and population control study. *Chinese Journal of Population Science*, (1), 34–39.

Chen, W. (2005). Migrant population and low fertility rate in Chinese cities. *Population Research, 29*(4), 79–83.

Chen, W., & Wu, L. (2006). Study on the relationship between migration and fertility in China. *Population Research, 30*(1), 13–20.

Chen, Y., & Ye, W. (2009). First birth interval of young female migrants and population control: Enlightenment from family survey of the floating population in Xiamen. *South China Population, 24*(4), 45–51.

Fu, C., Wang, W., & Zeng, X. (2012). Fertility change In China and its influencing factors: Analysis based on the sixth census. *South China Population, 27*(5), 1–10.

Fu, C., Zhang, L., & Li, Y. (2013). Characteristics of the changes of population fertility in China based on the sixth census. *Statistical Research, 30*(1), 68–75.

Gao, Y., & Wu, H. (2012). Impact of migration on average age at first marriage in Beijing. *Population Research, 36*(5), 58–68.

Guo, W. (2003). A preliminary analysis of the pattern of marriage and childbearing in China in the 1990s. *Population Journal*, (5), 18–21.

Guo, Z. (2010). Impacts of floating population on current fertility in China. *Population Research, 34*(1), 19–29.

Guo, Z., & Li, J. (2006). Research on birth interval in rural areas based on hierachical model. *Population Research, 30*(4), 2–11.

Jampaklay, A. (2006). How does leaving home affect marital timing? An event-history analysis of migration and marriage in Nang Rong, Thailand. *Demography, 43*(4), 711–725.

Jin, X., Peng, X., Li, S., Guo, Y., & Yang, X. (2005). Impacts of social network and integration on first marriage of female rural-urban immigrants: Evidence from survey in Pudong, Shanghai. *Population & Economics*, (5), 53–58 + 47.

Löfstedt, P., Ghilagaber, G., Shusheng, L., & Johansson, A. (2005). Changes in marriage age and first birth interval in Huaning County, Yunnan Province, PR China. *Southeast Asian Journal of Tropical Medicine and Public Health, 36*(5), 1329–1338.

Li, D., & Guo, Z. (2014). The fertility level of floating population in China: Based on the analysis of floating population dynamic monitoring data. *Chinese Journal of Population Science*, (3), 17–29 + 126.

Li, Y., & Jiang, Y. (2009). Analysis on the change of first birth interval of Chinese women since the 1980s. *Northwest Population Journal*, (3), 53–56.

Liang, T. (2016). The analysis of the birth intervals and its effecting factors of the rural-urban floating population: A case study of Shanghai city. *Population & Economics*, (5), 12–22.

Liu, H. (2014). Analysis on the age of first marriage of new generation floating population and its' determinant: Based on the floating population dynamic monitoring data. *Population and Development*, (5), 77–84.

Lu, J., & Wang, X. (2013). An analysis on the changes of marital status in China since the 1990s. *Social Sciences of Beijing*, (3), 62–72.

National Health Commission of China. (2016). *Report on China's Migrant population development*. Beijing: China Population Press.

Nath, D. C., Land, K. C., & Goswami, G. (1999). Effects of the status of women on the first-birth interval in Indian Urban Society. *Journal of Biosocial Science, 31*(1), 55–69.

Nenko, I., Hayward, A. D., & Lummaa, V. (2014). The effect of socio-economic status and food availability on first birth interval in a pre-industrial human population. *Proceedings of the Royal Society B Biological Sciences, 281*(1775), 20132319.

Ono, H. (2003). Women's economic standing, marriage timing, and cross-national contexts of gender. *Journal of Marriage and Family, 65*(2), 275–286.
Oppenheimer, V. K. (1988). A theory of marriage timing. *American Journal of Sociology, 94*(3), 563–591.
Rindfuss, R. R., & Morgan, S. P. (1983). Marriage, sex, and the first birth interval: The quiet revolution in asia. *Population & Development Review, 9*(2), 259.
Sedigheh, N. S., & Piri, N. (2012). The mean first birth interval and popular contraceptive method use before first pregnancy in women attending public health center of Ahvaz city, Iran 2010. *Life Science Journal-Acta Zhengzhou University Overseas Edition, 9*(4), 5815–5818.
Shafer, K., & Qian, Z. (2010). Marriage timing and educational assortative mating. *Journal of Comparative Family Studies, 41*(5), 661–691.
Shayan, Z., Ayatollahi, S. M., Zare, N., & Moradi, F. (2014). Prognostic factors of first birth interval using the parametric survival models. *Iranian Journal of Reproductive Medicine, 12*(2), 125–130.
Shi, Q., & Li, D. (2004). A comparative study on farmers' fertility behavior among different ethnic groups: From surveys of 418 peasant households in Hubei province. *Chinese Journal of Population Science,* (5), 58–66 + 82.
Silvey, R., & Elmhirst, R. (2003). Engendering social capital: Women workers and rural–urban networks in indonesia's crisis. *World Development, 31*(5), 865–879.
Singh, R., Tripathi, V., Kalaivani, M., Singh, K., & Dwivedi, S. N. (2012). Determinants of birth intervals in Tamil Nadu in India: Developing Cox hazard models with validations and predictions. *Revista Colombiana De Estadistica, 35*(2), 289–307.
Wang, F., & Yang, Q. (1996). Age at marriage and the first birth interval: The emerging change in sexual behavior among young couples in China. *Population & Development Review, 22*(2), 299.
Wu, H., Li, S., & Yue, Z. (2006). An analysis of fertility concept and behavior of rural migrants: Findings from a survey in Shenzhen. *Population Research, 30*(1), 61–68.
Xu, Q. (2015). Migration and its effect on the marriage timing of rural migrant workers: Gender differences. *Population & Economics,* (4), 39–51.
Zeng, Y. (1992). Estimation method of mean age at first marriage and average first birth interval based on census data and its application in the 4th data analysis. *Population & Economics,* (3), 3–8.
Zheng, Z. (1999). Analysis of first birth interval of Chinese women since the 1980s. *Population & Economics*, (2), 13–17.
Zheng, Z. (2000). Social-demographic influence on first birth interval in China, 1980–1992. *Journal of Biosocial Science, 32*(3), 315.

Chapter 10
Individual- and Community-Level Determinants of Contraceptive Behaviors in Young Female Migrants

Fang Tang

1 Introduction

According to the *Report on China's migrant population development 2017*, most Chinese internal migrants are new generations (post-80s). For example, the percentage of "post-80s" migrants rose from 50.0% in 2011 to 56.5% in 2016; the percentage of "post-90s" migrants increased from 14.5% in 2013 to 18.7% in 2016 (Wang, 2017). These new generations have more choices on family planning, but they also suffer from more reproductive diseases and unwanted pregnancy (Wang, Zhang, & Zhuang, 2019). Most new generations usually experience three basic processes: from rural to urban, from school to society, and from the single to the married (Ivanova, Rai, & Kemigisha, 2018). When new generations migrate into other places where they have no economic base, social acceptance, sense of belonging and cultural identity, they may face more challenges in specific life stages, such as marriage and birth (Ivanova et al., 2018), unprecedented reproductive health problems, and the contradiction between increasingly open-minded sexuality and family planning, especially after the Two-Child Policy conducted in 2015.

The Chinese central government released a detailed 10-year youth development plan *The Middle- and Long-term Youth Development Plan (2016–2025)* on 2017 April 13 (Xinhua, 2017), vowing better education, employment, and healthcare for Chinese young adults. One of the goals for youth development is that reproductive health information, education, counseling and access to safe, effective and affordable contraceptive and contraception technical services, as well as safe abortion, sexually transmitted diseases (STD) prevention and treatment services, should be available. Therefore, strengthening the management of reproductive health services for young

F. Tang (✉)
School of Health Sciences, Wuhan University, Wuhan, China
e-mail: tangfang@whu.edu.cn

P. Wang (ed.), *The Health Status of Internal Migrants in China*,
https://doi.org/10.1007/978-981-15-4415-6_10

female migrants is not only a requirement of *Healthy China 2030* (a national policy for constructing a healthier China), but also beneficial to improve the quality of reproductive health services and avoid unwanted pregnancy and abortion.

2 Literature Review

A suitable contraceptive behavior can avoid most reproductive diseases and unwanted pregnancy (Gu & Che, 2018). Because many women believe that ways of contraception do not affect postpartum recovery and breast-feeding, they usually choose convenient but unsafe contraceptive methods within 1 to 2 years after pregnancy, including safe contraception time, extramarital ejaculation and so forth (Cheng et al., 2018). After the universal Two-Child Policy, the rate of recurrent abortion for females with cicatrize pregnancy has increased, rising from 1.7 to 2.1%, because they are not forced by ligation and are more likely to experience unwanted pregnancy (Lv & Liang, 2018).

Evidence from other countries suggests that migrants usually use fewer health services than local residents, which leads to higher rates of unwanted pregnancy; one common explanation is that migrants are usually excluded by local policies and are socially isolated (Makenzius, Tydén, Darj, & Larsson, 2011; Rasch & Knudsen, 2008). However, the self-selection effect should not be ignored. Wandera et al. (2018) found that in Uganda, the contraceptive mode of American youth that received more education is different from that of their parents. After receiving more education, younger generations tend to delay their first sexual time, because they pursue equal partnership and usually choose a safer contraception method.

Numerous Chinese papers have been published, in which contraceptive behaviors are discussed using multiple statistical models. Using age-period-cohort (APC) and logistic regression models, Wang et al. (2019) found female migrants' contraceptive behavior changes with period, age and across successive cohorts, older women who experienced the One-Child Policy in their child-bearing period usually choose ligation and sterilization as their main contraceptive methods. Previously, younger female migrants left their hometown to have children in order to escape the family planning management and fines. Thus, factors that affect female's contraceptive behaviors do not result from the household registration policy, but from women's family support and some individual factors (household economic and cultural backgrounds) (Ding, Zhang, & Du, 2018; Liu, Li, Hong, & Yao, 2016; Zou & Liu, 2018). Women who are minority, with less education, less income and agricultural *hukou* are more likely to have long-acting and high-risk contraceptive behaviors. Furthermore, women who have boys or more than one child and with poor family economic conditions are more likely to choose long-acting contraceptive behaviors.

However, contextual effects on contraception have been discussed in prior studies. A study observes that household-level (Muslims), community-level (whether discussing family planning with friends or not) and contextual/supply-side (degree of remoteness of the village) factors are all essential prerequisites to determine female contraceptive choice (Saswata & Siddiqui, 2017). Similarity, Chinese internal migrants may be also influenced by living environments and policy implementations. For example, the community provides reproductive health education and free condoms for residents in China, which produce aggregate data, so it is necessary to examine the effect of these community interventions. Thus, the probability of type I errors in statistical test will increase when using a multivariate regression model, adding the personal factors, migration factors and community factors simultaneously to explore the influence factors of female reproductive health. Because people usually come together at the community level, it is necessary to consider the contextual effects on contraception.

The contraceptive choice of migrants is related to their migration behaviors. Once young female migrants leave their hometown, there are three stages (selection, adaption, disruption) for their psychological change. The selection means as a "self-selected" group, female migrants want to have a better life; compared with those women staying at hometown (usually rural areas), they may marry later and have more income (Arousell, Carlbom, Johnsdotter, & Essén, 2019; Ochako, Askew, Okal, Oucho, & Temmerman, 2016). When living in the city, they learn local cultures and lifestyles from the natives, which is considered the adaption. However, in this stage, women are facing some problems, because they are influenced by the cultural environment in different places, and it may change their choice of contraception. Thus, these stages are not isolated in the process of the whole migration. Healthy contraceptive behaviors in the early stage of reproductive life and appropriate spacing of pregnancies would significantly improve the health, education and labor force participation of women (Ochako et al., 2016).

3 Data and Methods

3.1 Data Source

This study used data from the China Migrants Dynamic Survey (CMDS) in Hubei Province between 2013 and 2017. CMDS is a large-scale nationally representative continuous cross-sectional survey. It collects information on migrants' demographic characteristics, living arrangements, health literacy, psychological health, and access to health care services. A Probability Proportionate to Size (PPS) sampling method is used to investigate migrants from different provinces. In CMDS, migrants aged 15–59 years and stayed in local areas for at least one month are investigated, they did not have local *hukou*.

In this chapter, we keep young female migrants who has married and under the age of 35, according to the definition of "Youth" released by the Chinese central government. Also select community-level include community reproductive education, family planning publicity column and family planning staff variables. Thus, a total of 5711 young female migrants were used in this study.

3.2 Data Analysis

The dependent variables in this chapter were contraceptive methods of migrant young women. In the questionnaire, the question "Do you want to have a baby within the next one year?" was firstly asked, and the response options included the following: '1 = yes' and '2 = no'; 'yes' means no contraceptive behavior, and 'no' means potential contraceptive behaviors. Subsequently, another question "which modern contraception is used primarily?" was asked, and the response options included the following: '1 = male sterilization', '2 = female sterilization', '3 = intrauterine contraceptive devices', '4 = subcutaneous implantations', '5 = injectable contraceptives', '6 = oral contraceptives', '7 = condoms', '8 = external contraceptives', '9 = intrauterine rings', '10 = safe contraception time', and '11 = external ejaculation'. Prior studies have proposed some classification methods on contraception. Ren (2008) proposed that male sterilization, female sterilization, intrauterine contraceptive device and subcutaneous implantation should be classified as medical-controlled contraception. By contrast, self-controlled contraceptive method consists of oral drugs, condoms, external drugs, and external ejaculation. Li, Wang, and Sun (2018) thought contraception could be divided into long- and short-acting types; short-acting contraceptive consists of oral contraceptive, condoms, and external use of drugs, while long-acting contraceptive consists of sterilization, intrauterine contraceptive device, and subcutaneous implantation. This study intended to divide contraceptive behaviors into three types. Low-risk long-acting contraception included female and male sterilization, intrauterine contraceptive device and subcutaneous implantation; low-risk short-acting contraception included injectable contraceptives, oral contraceptives, external contraceptives, male and female condom; high-risk contraception included safe contraception time, external ejaculation and not using any contraceptive method. Independent variables included individual level variables and community level variables. Individual level variables included age, religion (Han nationality and minority), number of children, number of boys, and time of migration, family monthly income, education (primary school or below, junior or senior high school, college or above), the Two-Child Policy (investigated before and investigated after).

Community level variables included number of family planning publicity columns within communities, supply of reproduction health education, number of family planning staffs. More information can be seen in Table 1.

3.3 Statistical Analysis

The aim of this chapter was to identify influencing factors of contraception mode. Due to the multilevel structure of the data, generalized linear model may yield biased estimations. Thus, a multilevel modeling technique was used, as it could adjust the standard errors of estimates for the clustering of observations within groups. In

Table 1 Descriptive information of variables used

Variable	Description
Individual-level	
Age	Continuous variable
Education	Primary school or below = 0, junior high school = 1, senior high school = 2, college or above = 3
Number of children	Continuous variable
Number of boys	Continuous variable
Ethnicity	Han nationality = 0, Minority = 1
Duration of migration	Continuous variable
Family monthly income	Log (income)
Two-Child Policy	Before Two-Child Policy year = 0, after Two-Child Policy year = 1
Community-level	
Number of family planning publicity column	Continuous variable
Free reproductive health services	No = 0, yes = 1
Number of staffs	Continuous variable

this chapter, high-risk contraception was used as the reference group, and a set of m−1 logistic regressions were performed for the rest two options. The multilevel multinomial model was specified as follows:

$$\log\left[\frac{P(m)}{P(3)}\right] = \beta_{0j(m)} + \beta_{1(m)}(ethnicity_i) + \beta_{2(m)}(boys_i) + \beta_{3(m)}(child_i) + \beta_{4(m)}(eduction_i) + \beta_{5(m)}(migrationduration_i) + \beta_{6(m)}(age_i) + \beta_{7(m)}(two - childpolicy_i) + \beta_{8(m)}(\log familyincome_i)$$

$$\beta_{0j(m)} = \gamma_{00(m)} + \gamma_{01(m)}\left(community_j\right) + \mu_{0(m)}$$

$$\beta_{2(m)} = \gamma_{20(m)} + \gamma_{02(m)}\left(community_j\right)$$

$$\beta_{3(m)} = \gamma_{30(m)} + \gamma_{03(m)}\left(community_j\right)$$

where $\beta_{0j(m)}$ (m ranged from 1 to 2) denoted two intercepts of the rest two categories. Accordingly, the left-hand side of the equation was the log-likelihood of adopting long-acting and short-acting contraceptive methods. The random effects (indicated by the subscript m) are measures of variations across different communities. For the analysis below, Model 1 represented the null model with no independent variable controlled for, it was used to understand the community-level unexplained variance on contraceptive behaviors that reflected using the intra-class correlation coefficient (ICC). Model 2 included individual-level variables to examine their independent effect on the choice of contraception. Community-level variables were included in Models 3 and 4 to investigate how community-level variables explained the community-level variation in contraceptive method, as well as the cross-level interaction effects between community- and individual-level factors. All analyses were performed using Stata 14.0 software.

4 Results

4.1 Descriptive Results

The number and percentage of sample characteristics based on individual-level and migrant characteristics for the pooled sample tabulated over the three contraception choices were presented in Table 2. A total of 5711 migrant respondents were analyzed in this study. The average age was 28.6 years old. Most young female migrants received junior or senior high school education (84.1%), a total of 12.0% females received college or above and only 3.9% females received primary school education or below. The majority (94.3%) of women had children, and more than half of the migrant females (58.4%) had one boy. In addition, average family income was 6651 Chinese Yuan (CNY) and average time duration of migration was 3.637 years. Nearly 51.0% females were using permanent methods, which was slightly higher than those using short-acting contraceptive methods (48.4%). Only 0.4% females were using high-risk contraceptive methods or having not contraceptive behavior. A total of 54.0% respondents were interviewed before the Two-Child Policy.

4.2 Results of Multilevel Multinomial Analysis

Table 3 presents the results of multilevel multinomial regression models. The ICC in null model (Model 1) shows that community-level factors were related to contraceptive behaviors. Models 2, 3 and 4 report the coefficients based on the multilevel multinomial analysis. Table 3 also shows the likelihood of long-acting and short-acting contraceptive behaviors relative to the likelihood of high-risk contraceptive behaviors.

ICC is expressed as the share of group-level random variance in total unobserved variance. Model 1 shows that $ICC_1 = 14.8\%$ and $ICC_2 = 15.2\%$, implying a significant community effect on contraceptive behaviors. Model 3 shows that the inclusion

Table 2 Socio-demographic and migrant characteristics among migrant young women (n = 5711)

Characteristics	n	Percentage (%) or M ± SD
Age	5711	28.639 ± 3.718
Education		
Primary school or below	225	3.9
Junior high school	3076	53.9
Senior high school	1726	30.2
College or above	684	12
Family monthly income	5711	6651.776 ± 4976.77
Ethnicity		
Minority	217	3.8
Han nationality	5494	96.2
Number of boys		
0	2376	41.6
1 and above	3335	58.4
Number of child		
0	325	5.7
1	3921	68.7
2 and above	1465	25.7
Duration of migration	5711	3.637 ± 3.067
Two-Child Policy		
Investigated before Two-Child Policy	3091	54.1
Investigated after Two-Child Policy	2620	45.9
Number of family planning publicity column		5.278 ± 6.925
Free reproductive health service education		
Yes	800	90
No	81	10
Number of staffs		1.763 ± 1.945

Note M: mean, SD: standard deviation

of community-level variables significantly reduced community-level random variance. ICC declined significantly from 15.2% to 9.4% (from Model I-2 to Model I-3) and from 18.6% to 9.0% (from Model II-2 to Model II-3). It indicates that the community-level variables used in this study can well explain the community-level variance of contraceptive behaviors.

Models I-2 and II-2 show that female migrants with one or more boys were more likely to have long-acting contraceptive behaviors ($\beta = 0.753$, OR = 2.123, $p < 0.001$), but were less likely to have short-acting contraceptive behaviors ($\beta = -0.574$, OR = 0.563, $p < 0.001$). The likelihood of choosing a long-acting contraceptive behavior increased significantly among female migrants who had one more children

Table 3 Multilevel-multinomial model estimates of contraceptive behaviors

	I high-risk versus long-acting				II high-risk versus short-acting			
	Model 1	Model 2	Model 3	Model 4	Model 1	Model 2	Model 3	Model 4
	β (SE)	β (SE)	β (SE)	β (SE)	β (SE)	β (SE)	β (SE)	β (SE)
Individual-level								
Intercept	−0.016(0.047)	1.187(0.724)	1.880(0.879)*	0.046(1.027)	−0.198(0.051)***	−1.670(0.715)*	−2.786(0.874)**	−1.199(1.026)
Ethnicity (ref: Han nationality)		0.506(0.198)*	0.447(0.229)	0.467(0.30)*		−0.425(0.193)*	−0.562(0.304)	−0.364(0.223)
Family income		−0.541(0.076)***	−0.536(0.090)***	−0.526(0.090)***		0.473(0.075)***	0.464(0.089)***	0.463(0.089)***
Number of boy (ref: no boy)		0.753(0.075)***	0.758(0.090)***	1.101(0.317)***		−0.574(0.074)***	−0.712(0.328)***	−0.901(0.315)***
Number of child		0.604(0.080)***	0.576(0.093)***	0.674(0.109)***		−0.214(0.079)***	−0.410(0.111)***	−0.442(0.114)***
Duration of migration		0.009(0.013)	−0.009(0.015)	0.010(0.018)		0.003(0.013)	0.007(0.015)	0.006(0.015)
Age		0.110(0.011)***	0.109(0.013)***	0.108(0.013)***		−0.110(0.010)***	−0.104(0.03)***	−0.105(0.013)***
Education (ref: primary school or below)								
Junior high		−0.604(0.197)***	−0.736(0.240)**	−0.727(0238)***		0.580(0.198)***	0.809(0.299)**	0.745(0.240)**
Senior high		−0.972(0.203)***	−1.132(0.249)***	−1.125(0.244)***		0.903(0.203)***	1.180(0.306)***	1.056(0.246)***
College or above		−2.134(0.235)***	−2.283(0.282)***	−2.276(0.282)***		1.989(0.230)***	2.354(0.349)***	2.131(0.277)***
Two−child Policy (ref: Before Two-Child Policy)		−0.913(0.097)***	−0.729(0.114)***	−0.124(0.321)***		1.119(0.096)***	1.106(0.097)***	0.354(0.323)
Community−level								
Number of family planning publicity column			−0.005(0.007)	0.036(0.017)			0.048(0.012)*	−0.043(0.017)*

(continued)

Table 3 (continued)

	I high-risk versus long-acting				II high-risk versus short-acting			
	Model 1	Model 2	Model 3	Model 4	Model 1	Model 2	Model 3	Model 4
Reproduction health education			−0.153(0.130)	1.274(0.467)**			0.493(0.175)**	−0.982(0.475)*
Number of staffs			−0.055(0.032)	−0.102(0.068)			0.010(0.004)	0.020(0.007)
Cross-level								
Family planning publicity column*boy				−0.025(0.013)*				0.033(0.013)*
Community reproduction health education*boy				−0.306(0.278)				0.255(0.275)
Community reproductive health education*two-child				−0.769(0.272)**				0.623(0.273)*
Random effects	$\sigma 1^2$				$\sigma 2^2$			
Estimates of intercept variance (SE) σz^2	0.755(0.091)	0.767(0.101)	0.586(0.100)	0.568(0.073)	0.910(0.104)	0.868(0.108)	0.572(0.141)	0.603(0.106)
−2LL	6558.237	5762.303	3955.134	3900.372	6471.857	5912.096	4070.382	3979.046
ICC	0.148	0.152	0.094	0.089	0.201	0.186	0.090	0.099
AIC	6562.237	5784.303	3981.134	3935.049	6475.857	5934.096	4096.382	4013.046
BIC	6575.234	5855.695	4060.737	4039.144	6488.854	6005.489	4175.984	4117.141

Note: *$p < 0.05$; **$p < 0.01$; ***$p < 0.001$
β coefficient, SE stand and error, -2LL -2log likelihood, ICC inter class correlation, AIC Akaike Inf ormation Criterion, BIC Bayesian Information Criterion

($\beta = 0.604$, OR = 1.829, $p < 0.001$) and who were older ($\beta = 0.110$, OR = 1.116, $p < 0.001$). By contrast, the results in Model II-2 show that the likelihood of choosing a short-acting contraceptive behavior increased significantly among female migrants who had one more children ($\beta = -0.214$, OR = 0.807, $p < 0.001$) and who were older ($\beta = -0.110$, OR = 0.896, $p < 0.001$). Female migrants who received free reproduction health education were more likely to have short-acting contraceptive behaviors ($\beta = 0.493$, OR = 1.637, $p < 0.01$). Besides, compared to the respondents who were interviewed before the Two-Child Policy, the odds of choosing short-acting contraceptive behaviors were more than three times higher (OR = 3.062, $p < 0.001$) for those who were interviewed after the Two-Child Policy. Furthermore, female migrants with higher education were more likely to have high-risk contraceptive behaviors (OR = 0.547, $p < 0.001$, OR = 0.378, $p < 0.001$, OR = 0.118, $p < 0.001$) but were less likely to have short-acting contraceptive behaviors (OR = 1.786, $p < 0.001$, OR = 2.467, $p < 0.001$, OR = 7.308, $p < 0.001$). However, no significant association between duration of migration and contraceptive behaviors was observed. It was strange that female migrants with more family income were less likely to choose high-risk contraceptive behaviors ($\beta = -0.541$, OR = 0.582, $p < 0.001$) but more likely to choose short-acting contraceptive behaviors ($\beta = 0.473$, OR = 1.605, $p < 0.001$).

As shown in Models I-3 and II-3, after controlling for community variables, the correlation between ethnicity and contraceptive behaviors became nonsignificant, but other variables did not change. Moreover, the respondents who lived in communities that provided free reproductive education were more likely to have short-acting contraceptive behaviors ($\beta = 0.493$, OR = 1.637, $p < 0.01$). Furthermore, if there were more family planning publicity columns in the community, female migrants were more likely to choose short-acting rather than high-risk contraceptive behaviors ($\beta = 0.048$, OR = 1.049, $p < 0.05$).

The interaction effects (cross-level interactions between community- and individual-level variables) were also examined in our analyses. The results in Models I-4 show that the interaction between number of family planning publicity column and number of boys ($\beta = -0.025$, OR = 0.975, $p < 0.05$), as well as between receiving reproduction health education and the Two-Child Policy ($\beta = -0.769$, OR = 0.537, $p < 0.01$), was statistically significant in high-risk versus long-acting contraceptive behaviors. Moreover, the results in Models II-4 show that the interaction between number of family planning publicity column and number of boys ($\beta = 0.033$, OR = 1.034, $p < 0.05$), as well as between receiving reproduction health education and the Two-Child Policy ($\beta = 0.623$, OR = 1.865, $p < 0.05$), was also statistically significant in high-risk versus short-acting contraceptive behaviors. Thus, living in communities with more family planning publicity columns, female migrants after the Two-Child policy were less likely to have long-acting contraceptive behaviors but more likely to have short-acting contraceptive behaviors. Similarly, living in communities that provided more reproduction health education, female migrants interviewed after the Two-Child Policy were less likely to have long-acting contraceptive behaviors but more likely to have short-acting contraceptive behaviors.

While the interaction effects between reproductive health education and the number of boys were statistically nonsignificant.

ICC is expressed as the share of group-level random variance in total unobserved variance. Model 1 shows that $ICC_1 = 14.8\%$ and $ICC_2 = 15.2\%$, implying a significant community effect on contraceptive behaviors. Model 3 shows that the inclusion of community-level variables significantly reduced community-level random variance. ICC declined significantly from 15.2% to 10.5% (from Model I-2 to Model I-3) and from 18.6% to 9.0% (from Model II-2 to Model II-3). It indicates that the community-level variables used in this study can well explain the community-level variance of contraceptive behaviors.

5 Discussion

This chapter found that ever since the Two-Child Policy went into effect, young female migrants in China have changed their contraceptive behaviors, after the Two-Child Policy, migrants were more likely to choose short-acting contraceptive behaviors compared to high-risk contraceptive behaviors. Furthermore, female migrants were less likely to choose long-acting contraceptive behaviors compared to high-risk contraceptive behaviors. It is observed that age, education, ethnicity, number of children, whether receiving reproductive health services, whether having a boy, and number of family planning publicity columns in the community were significantly related to female migrants' contraceptive behaviors. Especially, after the Two-Child Policy went into effect, Chinese migrant females would change their contraceptive behaviors to have a boy or a girl satisfied their aspiration. Without strict family planning supervision, Chinese female migrants are more vulnerable to premarital sex during reproductive period, as they have a lower level of education and health services utilization than local residents, which easily causes an unplanned pregnancy and sexually transmitted diseases (Gu & Che, 2018).

This study observes that duration of migration does not increase or reduce the probability of short-acting and high-risk contraceptive behaviors compared with that of long-acting contraceptive behaviors. There are some possible explanations. On one hand, young female migrants who leave their hometown longer or shorter and disrupt with their husbands presumably have more household autonomy and decision-making power in their households, this is actually a selection effect. On the other hand, condoms are easily accessible for female migrants no matter where they live in China. However, further study is required to establish a robust relationship.

Receiving reproductive health education and services is necessary for Chinese young female migrants. However, there are still 10% communities that cannot provide reproductive health services for migrant females, which means a lack of reproductive health services. A prior study has found a considerable influence of mass media exposure on adoption of modern temporary contraceptive methods in India and other developing countries (Kaggwa, Diop, & Storey, 2008). A recent study by Oliveira, Dias, and Padmadas (2014) also argues that family planning messages endorsed through mass media should be strengthened to inform couples of the effectiveness of reversible methods in birth spacing and its association with better maternal and child health outcomes, particularly among socio-economically vulnerable sections of society, and it is a good way to help reduce the incidence of AIDS.

Numerous prior studies have indicated a strong influence of women's education on their contraceptive behaviors or choices (Liu et al., 2016; Saswata & Siddiqui, 2017), which is in line with this study. Although some studies show that education is not associated with female's contraceptive choices in rural regions, they ignore that women in rural regions usually receive less education (Saswata & Siddiqui, 2017). Because well-educated female migrants are included (migrant females with senior high school or above accounts for over 30%), the significant relationship between education and contraceptive behaviors is well examined in this study.

The present study finds that female migrants of Han nationality are more likely to have modern temporary contraceptive behaviors (high-risk and short-acting behaviors), which is in line with the findings in many other studies (Ingleby, 2019; Oliveira et al., 2014). They find that minority female migrants are more likely to have long-acting contraceptive behaviors rather than short-acting contraceptive behaviors, and they are more likely to use condoms rather than sterilization. Because minority female migrants usually have a lower socioeconomic status than Han nationality female migrants, minority's preference for different contraceptive behaviors may attributable to childbearing policies, because minority females are allowed to have more children.

In concordance with the results of prior studies (Jayaraman, Mishra, & Arnold, 2007; Saswata & Begum, 2015), this chapter also shows that migrant young women in China usually switch over to permanent contraceptive behaviors from no contraceptive behavior after achieving their desired number of boys, which indicates the traditional preference for sons over daughters in Chinese culture. Moreover, this study finds that most young female migrants opt for permanent methods once their desired number of children is achieved. Many other studies (Ding et al., 2018; Oliveira et al., 2014; Saswata & Siddiqui, 2017) have also pointed out that owing children before have a decisive influence on the choice of permanent methods.

Whether providing health education and the number of family planning publicity columns are used as community-level factors to explain the community-level variance of female migrants' contraceptive behaviors. Although these two community-level factors cannot fully explain the variance of contraceptive behaviors across communities, significant effects of these two factors are observed. Other contextual factors excluded from the analysis should be examined in further studies.

According to the results of cross-level interaction analysis, when community's health education was provided, there was a significant difference in contraceptive behaviors before and after the implementation of the Two-Child policy. However, when community's health education was unprovided, there was a nonsignificant difference in contraceptive behaviors before and after the implementation of the Two-Child policy. It means the Two-Child Policy can affect the contextual effect of some other factors (not all) on the choice of contraception. Migrants' contraceptive behaviors will change and improve by receiving reproductive health education and publicity columns from the community, so the government should enhance the publicity of avoiding high-risk contraceptive behaviors and pay more attention to females who have a child but without using any contraception, especially young female migrants with junior or lower educational attainment.

This study still has some limitations. First, because of the short time interval between the surveys, a cross-sectional analysis is used, which does not help establish a causal relationship. Second, because no other variables that are found to be related to contraceptive behaviors (e.g. family members' perceptions of contraceptive behaviors, whether the community purchased appropriate pills) in this study, the influence of factors included may be somewhat overestimated. Finally, this study is based on a small-scale survey in Hubei Province, so it is hard to be generalized. In conclusion, both the variables at the individual level and at the community level affect the migrants' choice of contraceptive measures, the community should increase the propaganda on reproductive health, so as to promote a rational contraception of migrant women.

References

Arousell, J., Carlbom, A., Johnsdotter, S., & Essén, B. (2019). Are 'low socioeconomic status' and 'religiousness' barriers to minority women's use of contraception? A qualitative exploration and critique of a common argument in reproductive health research. *Midwifery, 75,* 59–65.

Cheng, L., Di, W., Ding, Y., Fan, G., Gu, X., Hao, M., & Jin, H. et al. (2018). Chinese expert consensus on clinical application of female contraceptive methods. *Reproductive and Developmental Medicine, 2*(4), 208–223.

Ding, Z., Zhang, Y., & Du, S. (2018). Patterns and determinants of contraceptive use among married migrant women in China. *Population Research, 42*(4), 27–38.

Gu, X., & Che, Y. (2018). The enlightenment of big data on induced abortion and contraception to the family planning work in China after the relaxation of the family planning policy. *Chinese Journal of Practical Gynecology and Obstetrics, 34*(1), 46–51.

Ingleby, D. (2019). Moving upstream: changing policy scripts on migrant and ethnic minority health. *Health Policy, 123*(9), 809–817.

Ivanova, O., Rai, M., & Kemigisha, E. (2018). A systematic review of sexual and reproductive health knowledge, experiences and access to services among refugee, migrant and displaced girls and young women in Africa. *International Journal of Environmental Research and Public Health, 15*(8), e1583.

Jayaraman, A., Mishra, V., & Arnold, F. (2007). *The effect of family size and composition on fertility desires, contraceptive adoption, and method choice in south Asia*. DHS Working Paper.

Kaggwa, E. B., Diop, N., & Storey, D. (2008). The role of individual and community normative factors: a multilevel analysis of contraceptive use among women in union in Mali. *International Perspectives on Sexual and Reproductive Health, 34*(2), 79–88.

Li, J., Wang, T., & Sun, Z. (2018). From health advantage to health disadvantage: the epidemiological paradox in rural migrants. *Population Research, 42*(6), 46–60.

Liu, Z., Li, J., Hong, Y., & Yao, L. (2016). Reproductive health service utilization and social determinants among married female rural-to-urban migrants in two metropolises, China. *Journal of Huazhong University of Science and Technology, 36*(9), 904–909.

Lv, Y., & Liang, Q. (2018). Investigation and analysis of influencing factors of recurent induced abortion rate among floating population women of childbearing age in a district of Shanghai before and after the Two-Child Policy. *Chinese Journal of Clinical Medicine, 25*(4), 668–670.

Makenzius, M., Tydén, T., Darj, E., & Larsson, M. (2011). Repeat induced abortion: a matter of individual behaviour or societal factors? A cross-sectional study among Swedish women. *European Journal of Contraception and Reproductive Health Care, 16*(5), 369–377.
Ochako, R., Askew, I., Okal, J., Oucho, J., & Temmerman, M. (2016). Modern contraceptive use among migrant and non-migrant women in Kenya. *Reproductive Health, 13,* e67.
Oliveira, I. T. D., Dias, J. G., & Padmadas, S. S. (2014). Dominance of sterilization and alternative choices of contraception in India: An appraisal of the socioeconomic impact. *Plos One, 9*(1), e86654.
Rasch, V., & Knudsen, L. (2008). Reply to induced abortion in Denmark: Effect of socio-economic situation and country of birth. *European Journal of Public Health, 18*(5), 540–540.
Saswata, G., & Begum, S. (2015). Influence of son preference on contraceptive method mix: Evidences from "two bengals". *Asian Population Studies, 11*(3), 1–16.
Saswata, G., & Siddiqui, M. Z. (2017). Role of community and context in contraceptive behaviour in rural west bengal, India: A multilevel multinomial approach. *Journal of Biosocial Science, 49*(1), 48–68.
Wandera, S. O., Kwagala, B., & Odimegwu, C. (2018). Intimate partner violence and current modern contraceptive use among married women in Uganda: A cross-sectional study. *Pan African Medical Journal, 30,* e85.
Wang, P. (2017). *Report on China' migrant population development.* Beijing: China Population Publshing House.
Wang, Z., Zhang, J., & Zhuang, Y. (2019). Analyses on migrants' contraceptive mix change in China during 2011−2017. *Population Journal, 45*(9), 5–17.
Xinhua. (2017). China unveils 10-year plan for youth development. Retrieved from http://english.www.gov.cn/policies/latest_releases/2017/04/14/content_281475626290850.htm.
Zou, Y., & Liu, H. (2018). Evolution of contraception mix in China, 2010−2016. *Population Research, 42*(5), 3–16.

Chapter 11
How Does the Education of Migrants Influence Their Accompanying Elderly Parents' Health?

Junfeng Jiang

1 Introduction

In the setting of social economy transition in China, the number of internal migrants has been booming with industrialization and urbanization, reaching 244 million in 2017 (National Bureau of Statistics, 2018), and most of them are young labors from rural China. In this process, family migration has emerged and become more and more popular. In order to take care of their juniors and lead a comfortable life in their later years, many elderly people choose to migrate with their children. However, migrant seniors are usually unable to have access to equivalent healthcare services as local urban elderly, for the supporting facilities in urban areas are inadequate. Most migrant seniors have no income and live with and depend on their children, so there are more direct contacts among these migrants. However, limited studies have discussed this special population, and their health-related issues have been ignored in most cases (Nie, Pan, Sun, & Bao, 2017).

Some evidence suggests that a shorter distance of the residence between the elderly and their children is more beneficial for the later to support their parents (Ding, You, & Wei, 2017; Zhang & Li, 2004b). This kind of support matters for old-age endowment (Hu, 2017). For example, children's economic and emotional support to their parents can not only improve their parents' daily care, but also improve their health (Zhang & Li, 2004a). For internal migrants, their education plays an important and special role in a similar way in this process. On one hand, education is a kind of human capital with great economic values (Zhang, Zhao, Park, & Song, 2005) and provides a basis and possibility of intergenerational economic support for migrant seniors. On the other hand, as an important way of socialization, education has an important impact on individual's behavioral patterns and values (Yuan, 2010). From this point of view, the education of migrants is closely associated with the

J. Jiang (✉)
School of Health Sciences, Wuhan University, Wuhan, China
e-mail: jiang0111@whu.edu.cn

P. Wang (ed.), *The Health Status of Internal Migrants in China*,
https://doi.org/10.1007/978-981-15-4415-6_11

number and quality of intergenerational emotional support for their accompanying parents. Therefore, the education of migrants may have a significant impact on their accompanying elderly parents' health. Given the instrumental and emotional support that results from education, this study aims to examine how the education of migrants influences the health of their elderly parents who migrate with them, and discusses the moderating effect of some economic factors in this process.

2 Literature Review and Research Hypotheses

The causal association between education and health has been widely discussed for a long time (Damon & Healther, 2013). According to the Health Production Theory, education can promote health by increasing the investment in health capital (Grossman, 1972; Ross & Wu, 1995). Education may promote health in multiple ways. On one hand, education can promote health through increasing income or improving socioeconomic status (SES) (Ross & Wu, 1995; Wu, 2009). On the other hand, a higher level of education produces more health knowledge and a higher level of health consciousness, so individuals with high-level education are more likely to choose a healthy lifestyle and make better use of healthcare services to prevent or cure diseases (Mak, Woo, Bowling, Wong, & Chau, 2011; Ross & Wu, 1995; Yamashita & Brown, 2017).

However, previous studies on education and health mainly examine how individuals' education influences their own health. When education and health outcomes belong to two different but related subjects, does the association between them still exist? Numerous studies suggest that education has the feature of externality (Cui, 2003; Miguel & Kremer, 2004), for one's education can influence the well-being or health of surrounding persons. Since family is an independent unit of life and production that consists of blood or marriage relationship, there should be strong ties among family members (Fei, 2013). Thus, the externality of education on health mainly appears between family members.

The externality of education on health between family members can be divided into three modes: influence between peers, influence from parents to their children, and influence from children to their parents, and all three modes are proved to be possible. For example, for the influence between peers, evidence indicates that individuals with a higher level of education have a beneficial impact on the health behavior and health outcome of their spouse (Bosma, Appels, Sturmans, Grabauskas, & Gostautas, 1995; Jaffe, Eisenbach, Neumark, & Manor, 2006; Monden, Lenthe, Graaf, & Kraaykamp, 2003). For the second mode, some evidence indicates that if parents have a higher level of education, their children will be healthier in their childhood (Chen, 2011), and if a father have a higher level of education, his children are more likely to be healthy in their later years (Cheng, Zhang, & Shen, 2015). For the last mode, some evidence also suggests that offspring's education usually has a positive effect on their parents' health (Jiang, 2019; Wu, 2009). The externality of education in the last mode provides a useful theoretical perspective for the present study.

Accordingly, it was assumed that similar externality of education may also exist in Chinese internal migrants: there should be a positive association between the education of migrants and their accompanying elderly parents' health. If migrants had a higher level of education, they would have access to economic resources, healthcare services, social network resources and health knowledge more easily. Therefore, the benefit of these resources might be translated into the health of their parents through intergenerational support. Accordingly, it is hypothesized that:

Hypothesis 1: *The higher level of education that migrants own, the better health that their elderly parents would gain.*

Evidence from multilevel studies suggests that health is not only influenced by individual factors, but also affected by contextual factors (Vettore & Aqeeli, 2016). Living in a context with a developed economy and more healthcare services, individuals can get a better living condition and more high-quality healthcare resources, so they tend to be healthier (Li, 2004). The completeness of healthcare system and the access to healthcare resources are greatly determined by the level of regional socioeconomic development (Sheng & Tian, 2015). In other words, when the ability to acquire healthcare resources is equal, the acquirement of healthcare resources is restricted by the amount of resources itself. In a more developed society, healthcare resources are usually richer, so the following consequence usually appears: individuals with a higher level of education can get healthcare services more conveniently, but individuals with a lower level of education are more likely to bear the detrimental impact of such developed economy. Accordingly, it is hypothesized that:

Hypothesis 2a: *The higher the level of macro social economic development, the better health the migrant seniors would gain.*

Hypothesis 2b: *The positive effect of migrants' education on the health of their accompanying elderly parents is larger in areas with a high-level macro social economy than in those with a low-level macro social economy.*

Individuals' health is influenced not only by the economic support but also by emotional support they can get (Zhang & Li, 2004a). It is recognized that the emotional solace from children can benefit their elderly parents' health (Mu, 2004). Intergenerational emotional support is mostly expressed as intergenerational affective interaction and affective company, which are both related to intergenerational interaction. In contemporary China, generation difference emerges to be larger and has gradually become an obstacle of intergenerational interaction (Zhou, 2017). Generation difference mainly means the difference in ideology and value between old and new generations (Zhou, 2017), so the generation difference in education is an important reflection of it. A larger generation difference in education usually means fewer proper communications, which may reduce the intergenerational affective support from children to their parents. Accordingly, it is hypothesized that:

Hypothesis 3: *The larger the generation difference in education between migrants and their elderly parents, the poorer health the latter would have.*

Education can promote health through the production of more income or higher SES (Ross & Wu, 1995; Wu, 2009). Since children's economic support is an important promoting factor of their parents' health (Zhang & Li, 2004b), the disparity in economic capability of migrants with similar levels of education may lead to disparities in the supply of intergenerational economic support. Therefore, income may reduce the disparity in the health return of education (Schnittker, 2004). In other words, there may be a substitution effect, and with the help of high-level income, migrants with less education can also help promote their parents' health well. Accordingly, it is hypothesized that:

Hypothesis 4: *The positive effect of migrants' education on their elderly parents' health will be smaller if they have more personal or family income.*

Accordingly, this study uses data from a nationally respresentative survey to examine the above hypotheses.

3 Data and Methods

3.1 Data Source and Sample Matching

The data we used were from the China Migrants Dynamic Survey (CMDS) in 2015 and *China Statistical Yearbook 2016*. The National Health and Family Planning Commission of China has conducted CMDSs covering all provincial administrative regions every year in mainland China since 2009. A stratified multi-stage probability-proportional-to-size sampling (PPS) method was used to ensure the national representativeness of the data. During 2009–2014, migrants aged 15–59 years and lived in local place for no less than one month with no local *hukou*[1] were investigated. In CMDS 2015, migrant seniors aged 60 years or older were surveyed, which provided valuable data for this study.

Since not all migrant seniors investigated were the parents of younger respondents in this survey, a filtration was conducted. First, respondents from Hong Kong, Macao, Taiwan and other foreign countries were excluded, and only respondents in mainland China were included. Second, two questions which are about the relationship between respondents and trailing migrant seniors were used to find out whether the migrant seniors were the natural parents or parents-in-law of younger migrant respondents. Finally, 4682 valid samples were obtained. Since the natural parents and parents-in-law were coded the same in the questionnaire, they were both considered as migrants' parents in this study.

[1]Three categories of people are excluded: (1) one of the couple is not migrant; (2) parents are migrants but children are not migrants; (3) soldiers and students.

3.2 *Variables*

3.2.1 Explanatory Variables

The education of migrants and the generation difference in education were used as two explanatory variables. In the questionnaire, the coding of migrants' education ranges from 1 to 7, which denotes illiteracy, primary school, junior high school, senior high school, junior college, college or above in order. Thus, migrants' education was recoded as four dummy variables (see Table 1), and the education of primary school or below was used as the reference group. For the generation difference in education, the education of interviewed migrants was used to subtract the education of their elderly parents, and then the absolute value of the original difference obtained was used as the generation difference in education. Certainly, most migrants had a higher level of education than their elderly parents who migrated with them.

3.2.2 Dependent Variable

The question "what is your health status?" was used to measure the self-rated health (SRH) of migrants' elderly parents. The response options included the following: "1 = very poor, 2 = poor, 3 = good, 4 = very good" (see Table 1). Since the interaction effect can be explained easier in an ordinary least squares (OLS) model, SRH was treated as a continuous variable in this study. Numerous studies propose that this strategy can yield similar results compared to an ordinal logistic regression model (Zheng, Yang, & Land, 2011).

3.2.3 Moderating Variables

Three economic factors were used as moderating variables. At the individual level, migrant's personal monthly income and family monthly income were used, and the unit was Chinese Yuan (CNY). The value of zero was recoded into one and then a natural logarithm transform was performed to make them follow a normal distribution. At the macro level, the gross domestic product (GDP) per capita at the province level was used, and the unit was also CNY.

3.2.4 Control Variables

Some characteristics of migrant seniors were used as control variables, including sex, age, *hukou*, education, range of migration, duration of migration, daily exercise time, number of local friends, and economic source. Details are displayed in Table 1.

Table 1 Basic information of variables used

Variables	Recoding	%	M/SD	Unit
Control variables				
Sex	Male = 0 Female = 1	46.1 53.9		
Age			67.378/6.833	
Hukou	Rural = 0 Urban = 1	28.4 71.6		
Education	Illiteracy Primary school Junior high school Senior high school or above	27.4 44.5 19.5 8.6		
Range of migration	Trans-province = 0 Inter-province = 1	44.7 55.3		
Duration of migration[a]	Continuous variable		5.650/5.743	Year
Daily exercise time	Continuous variable		64.375/47.219	Minute
Local friends number	Count variable		7.091/9.390	
Economy source	Income Retirement pension Family members Others	12.4 23.4 51.0 13.2		
Explanatory variables				
Education	Primary school or below Junior high school Senior high school Junior college College or above	15.8 44.4 20.3 10.8 8.7		
Generation difference in education			1.471/1.048	
Moderating variables				
Personal income	Continuous variable		8.199/0.917	
Family income	Continuous variable		8.803/0.653	
GDP per capita	Continuous variable		52,676/2.470	CNY
Dependent variable				
SRH	Very poor = 1 Poor = 2 Healthy = 3 Very healthy = 4	2.3 10.1 40.2 47.4		

Note M: mean, SD: standard deviation, CNY: Chinese Yuan

[a]In China, the Spring Festival is an important time point for internal migrants. Because of this festival, most internal migrants go back home in January and leave their hometown in February. Thus, the year between one respondent left its hometown and the investigation year was used as the duration of migration

3.3 Methods

Hierarchical linear model (HLM), also called multilevel model or mixed effects model, allows and can address the correlation of outcomes across subgroups (J. Wang, Xie, & Jiang, 2008). In this study, all of the respondents came from 31 provinces, so the data could be considered multilevel and might suffer the problem of interclass correlation. Therefore, this study used a two-level multilevel model, including the individual and province levels, to address potential problem of interclass correlation. The model specification is as follows:

Level-1 model:

$$\begin{aligned} Health_{ij} = & \beta_{0j} + \sum(\beta_k * edu_{ki}) + \sum\left(\beta_p * edu_{ki} * family\,income_i\right) \\ & + \sum\left(\beta_q * edu_{ki} * personal\,income_i\right) + \sum(\beta_m * x_i) + e_{ij} \end{aligned}$$

Level-2 model:

$$\beta_{0j} = \gamma_{00} + \alpha_{00} * GDP_j + u_{0j}$$

$$\beta_k = \gamma_{k0} + \alpha_{k0} * GDP_j$$

where $Health_{ij}$ denoted the health of individual i in province j; β_{0j} meant the intercept, including the fixed intercept γ_{00} and the random parameter u_{0j}, and α_{00} was the coefficient of GDP per capita in province j; edu_{ki} denoted the kth educational level of individual i, γ_{k0} was the kth fixed coefficient and α_{k0} denoted the kth interaction coefficient between GDP per capita and education; $\sum\left(\beta_p * edu_{ki} * family\,income_i\right)$ denoted the interaction between education and family income, and $\sum\left(\beta_q * edu_{ki} * personal\,income_i\right)$ meant the interaction between education and personal income; $\sum(\beta_m * x_i)$ denoted the fixed effect of other covariates at the individual level; e_{ij} was the random error that followed a normal distribution.

The endogeneity problem in the causality between education and health has been widely discussed. In this study, migrant seniors' better health might increase family income and help their children get high-quality education. On the other hand, there might be some confounding factors in above multilevel models, which influenced not only migrant seniors' health but also their children's education attainment, so the estimation might be biased and needs to be re-examined. Accordingly, the propensity score matching (PSM) approach was used to address these potential endogeneity problems (Hu, 2015) so as to yield the causal effect of migrants' education on their accompanying elderly parents' health in this study. Because migrants' education, the treatment, was an ordinal variable, the inverse probability of treatment weighting (IPTW) method (Cao, Durden, & Mark, 2009; Hong, 2015) was used to address potential endogeneity problems, and the average treatment effect on the treated (ATT) was estimated in this study. As confounding factors should be both related to treatment and outcome, family income, accompanying parents' education, accompanying parents' duration of migration, accompanying parents' range of migration and generation difference in education were selected as confounding factors.

In this study, SAS 9.4 was used to perform the above models, and $\alpha = 0.1$ was set as the statistical significance level.

4 Results

4.1 Moderating Effect of Family and Personal Income

The effect of migrants' education on their accompanying elderly parents' health and the moderating effect of family and personal income were first examined. Table 2 shows that the interclass correlation coefficient (ICC) was 0.056, indicating that 5.6% of the variation of accompanying elderly parents' health could be explained at the province level ($p < 0.001$). Model 2 shows that migrants' education was positively associated with their accompanying elderly parents' health. Compared with the migrants with primary school education or below, migrants with junior college education had the largest positive effect on their accompanying parents' health. Furthermore, the positive effect of migrants' education on their accompanying elderly parents' health was smaller if migrants had a higher level of personal income, and this moderating effect was significant in migrants with junior college education or above. Thus, Hypothesis 4 is partly supported.

4.2 Effect of Generation Difference in Education

In Model 4, accompanying elderly parents' characteristics and behaviors were controlled for, and more education of migrants was still related to their accompanying elderly parents' better health, but migrants with senior high school education had the largest health effect. In Model 5, the generation difference in education was added, but it was not statistically related to migrant seniors' health, for there might be a multicollinearity issue among the three education-related variables. Therefore, migrant seniors' education was deleted in Model 6, and the results indicated that a higher level of migrants' education was related to their accompanying elderly parents' better health, and a larger generation difference in education resulted in poorer health of their accompanying elderly parents. Thus, Hypotheses 1 and 3 are supported.

Table 2 Effect of migrants' education on their accompanying elderly parents' health: moderating effect of income

Variables	Model 1		Model 2		Model 3	
	β	SE	β	SE	β	SE
Fixed effects						
Intercept	3.303***	0.034	3.328***	0.024	3.344***	0.024
Education of migrants (ref: edu0)						
edu1			0.162***	0.034	0.143***	0.037
edu2			0.271***	0.039	0.249***	0.042
edu3			0.281***	0.047	0.278***	0.051
edu4			0.191***	0.053	0.257***	0.063
Family income			0.147***	0.024	0.159***	0.024
Personal income			0.024	0.015	0.020	0.016
edu1*Family income					0.041	0.069
edu2*Family income					−0.118	0.079
edu3*Family income					−0.059	0.089
edu4*Family income					−0.015	0.107
edu1*Personal income					−0.058	0.043
edu2*Personal income					0.006	0.055
edu3*Personal income					−0.123*	0.057
edu4*Personal income					−0.228*	0.089
Random effects-variance component						
Province	0.031***	0.009	0.014**	0.005	0.014**	0.005
ICC	0.056		0.028		0.027	
BIC	10391		8786		8790	
n	4682		4076		4076	

Note ***$p < 0.001$, **$p < 0.01$, *$p < 0.05$, ^$p < 0.1$. *β* coefficient, *SE* standard error, *edu0* primary school or below, *edu1* junior high school, *edu2* senior high school, *edu3* junior college, *edu4* college or above, *ICC* inter-class correlation, *BIC* Bayesian Information Criterion

4.3 Effect of Macro Socioeconomic Development

Table 4 suggests that provincial GDP per capita not only had a positive effect on older adults' health, but also had a negative moderating effect on the association between migrants' education and their accompanying elderly parents' health. However, living in a more developed region reduced the positive effect of migrants' education on their accompanying elderly parents' health only when the migrants owned a high-level education. Thus, Hypothesis 2a is supported and Hypothesis 2b is not supported.

Table 3 Migrants' education, generation difference in education and migrant seniors' health

Variables	Model 4		Model 5		Model 6	
	β	SE	β	SE	β	SE
Intercept	3.314***	0.023	3.314***	0.023	3.314***	0.023
Self-factors						
Sex	0.030	0.021	0.030	0.021	0.034^	0.021
Age	−0.013***	0.002	−0.013***	0.002	−0.014***	0.002
Hukou	−0.016	0.028	−0.016	0.028	−0.015	0.028
Education (ref: illiteracy)						
primary school	0.078**	0.026	0.050	0.034		
junior high school	0.131***	0.034	0.076	0.056		
senior high school or above	0.122**	0.046	0.046	0.075		
Range of migration	0.100***	0.024	0.099***	0.024	0.098***	0.024
Duration of migration	−0.002	0.002	−0.002	0.002	−0.002	0.002
Daily exercise time	0.002***	0.000	0.002***	0.000	0.002***	0.000
Local friends number	0.005***	0.001	0.005***	0.001	0.005***	0.001
Economy sources (ref: others)						
income	0.256***	0.052	0.257***	0.052	0.256***	0.052
retirement pension	0.031	0.038	0.030	0.038	0.026	0.037
other family members	0.029	0.031	0.028	0.031	0.028	0.031
Education of migrants (ref: primary school or below)						
junior high school	0.104***	0.031	0.135***	0.039	0.162***	0.032
senior high school	0.175***	0.037	0.234***	0.060	0.283***	0.042
junior college	0.162***	0.045	0.250**	0.082	0.315***	0.054
college or above	0.118*	0.052	0.236*	0.107	0.317***	0.066
Generation difference in education			−0.032	0.025	−0.053***	0.014
Random effects-variance component						
Province	0.013**	0.004	0.013**	0.004	0.013**	0.004
ICC	0.028		0.028		0.028	
BIC	9789		9793		9782	
n	4682		4682		4682	

Note ***$p<0.001$, **$p<0.01$, *$p<0.05$, ^$p<0.1$. β coefficient, *SE* standard error, *ICC* inter-class correlation, *BIC* Bayesian Information Criterion

4.4 Robust Analysis: Based on PSM

Table 5 shows that the estimated effect of migrants' education on their accompanying elderly parents' health in PSM is similar to those in multilevel models in Tables 2, 3 and 4. Although the estimated effect of migrants' education on their accompanying

Table 4 Migrants' education and their accompanying elderly parents' health: effect of macro socioeconomic development

Variables	Model 7		Model 8		Model 9	
	β	SE	β	SE	β	SE
Intercept	3.310***	0.026	3.317***	0.026	3.319***	0.026
Education of migrants (ref: primary school or below)						
junior high school	0.202***	0.032	0.197***	0.032	0.261***	0.033
senior high school	0.324***	0.037	0.317***	0.037	0.449***	0.041
junior college	0.358***	0.043	0.357***	0.045	0.556***	0.052
college or above	0.322***	0.049	0.380***	0.056	0.665***	0.067
Generation difference in education					−0.106***	0.014
GDP per capita	0.035**	0.011	0.036**	0.011	0.035**	0.011
Cross-level interaction effects						
GDP*junior high school			−0.017	0.015	−0.017	0.015
GDP*senior high school			−0.012	0.017	−0.013	0.017
GDP*junior college			−0.025	0.018	−0.026	0.018
GDP*college or above			−0.047*	0.019	−0.049**	0.019
Random effects-variance component						
Province	0.017**	0.006	0.016**	0.005	0.017**	0.006
ICC	0.031		0.030		0.032	
BIC	10306		10326		10275	
n	4682		4682		4076	

Note ***$p < 0.001$, **$p < 0.01$, *$p < 0.05$, ^$p < 0.1$. β coefficient, *SE* standard error, *GDP* Gross Domestic Product, *ICC* inter-class correlation, *BIC* Bayesian Information Criterion

elderly parents' health is smaller in Model 10 than in Model 11, they actually show consistent results. That is to say, the more education the migrants received, the better health their accompanying elderly parents would gain. Therefore, Hypothesis 1 is supported again.

5 Discussion and Conclusions

Using data from a nationally representative survey in 2015, this study examined the effect of migrants' education on the health of their accompanying elderly parents

Table 5 Migrants' education and their accompanying elderly parents' health: based on PSM

Variables	Model 10		Model 11	
	ATT	Robust SE	ATT	Robust SE
Intercept	3.246***	0.092	3.185***	0.064
Migrants' education (ref: primary school or below)				
junior high school	0.079	0.094	0.122^	0.069
senior high school	0.163^	0.095	0.307***	0.069
junior college	0.184^	0.101	0.335**	0.126
college or above	0.318^	0.168	0.727***	0.085
n	4679		4534	

Note ***$p < 0.001$, **$p < 0.01$, *$p < 0.05$, ^$p < 0.1$. *ATT* average treatment effect on the treated, *SE* standard error. All estimations pasted the balance test, and the standard bias of almost all covariates was less than 0.10 after matching (Hong, 2015). Since the valid sample size within common support was too small when adding accompanying parents' education and generation difference in education into one model at the same time, we respectively added them into two models. The confounding factors in Model 10 were family income, accompanying parents' education, accompanying parents' duration of migration and accompanying parents' range of migration, while in Model 11 they were family income, accompanying parents' duration of migration, accompanying parents' range of migration and the generation difference in education

in China. The moderating effects of personal income, family income and GDP per capita, as well as the effect of generation difference in education, were also examined.

First, this study demonstrates that there is a robust positive association between migrants' education and their accompanying elderly parents' health, which supports the externality of education. The mechanism why migrants' education influences their accompanying elderly parents' health can be summarized into four points. First, migrants' education may influence their accompanying elderly parents' health by improving their ability to obtain physical resources. In other words, individuals with a higher level of education are more likely to obtain a better occupational status or more income in labor market. Therefore, their accompanying elderly parents can get better economic guarantee and more healthcare resources and are more likely to be healthy. Second, taking the generation difference in education into account, the positive effect of migrants' education on their accompanying elderly parents' health becomes stronger. It demonstrates that emotional barrier is a key risk factor that reduces the positive externality of migrants' education on their accompany elderly parents' health, which suggests the importance of intergenerational emotional support in this process. Third, a higher level of migrants' education means more knowledge about health; on the basis of intergenerational feedback (Zhou, 2017), accompanying elderly parents can learn some knowledge about health more or less from their children and become healthier. Finally, the social expectation mechanism may also matters. In modern China, one's scholastic achievement is still an important expectation of his/her parents. A higher level of education usually means a successful life, so it can fulfill parents' social expectation to a great extent (Wang & Shi, 2014). If an individual gets a higher level of education, his/her parents will feel more valued and more sense of achievement in their life (Willis, 1982). Thus, a higher level of migrants' education results in a better health status of their accompanying elderly parents.

Second, some evidence from peer groups suggests that the educational difference between couples negatively relates to their health (Vernon & Buffler, 1988). Thus, the generation difference in education should be noticed. Previous studies have demonstrated that the affective interaction across different generations is a protective factor for older adults' health (Zhang & Li, 2004a). A smaller generation difference in education can reduce communication barriers, thus benefiting accompanying elderly parents' health. China has witnessed a profound but tortuous development over the past several decades, the education difference between Chinese middle-young people and the elderly is relatively large. Education is an important way to shape our values and produce generation differences (Zhou, 2017), so a large generation difference in education has a non-ignorable detrimental effect on elderly people's health. On the other hand, intergenerational emotional support from migrant offspring with a higher level of education is more likely to be replaced by economic support (Fan, 2016). If offspring owns a higher level of education, the generation difference in education is probable to be larger, which may make the estimation on the effect of migrants' education on their accompanying parents' health biased.

Finally, the positive effect of migrants' education on their accompanying elderly parents' health is moderated by income or economic factors. The positive effect of migrants' education on their accompanying elderly parents' health is smaller if the migrants have more income, and the positive effect of migrants' education on their accompanying eldely parents' health is also smaller in a high-level macro social economy than in a low-level macro economy. Living in a developed region, migrants usually face more social competitions and stress. As a higher level of education usually means more social expectations, migrants with a higher level of education are more likely to experience this kind of stress. They should earn more money, at a cost of increased working hours and less rest time. Thus, they have less time to communicate with their parents, which is a risk factor for the health of their accompanying elderly parents.

Accordingly, some suggestions on how to improve the health of older migrants in China are proposed. (1) Increasing the investment in educational development and improving the educational level and literacy of all citizens. We should especially promote the education of internal migrants to provide more economic and health knowledge resources for their accompanying elderly parents' health in China. (2) Maintaining the development of regional economy so as to provide sufficient socioeconomic and healthcare resources support. The development of productivity is the fundamental way to address the health problem of migrant seniors, which can increase migrants' income and enrich healthcare resources. (3) Attaching more attention to specific groups of migrant seniors. For example, migrant seniors with few local friends should be encouraged to engage in social activities to rebuild their social networks actively. (4) Increasing intergenerational communications and emotional support from the offspring. (5) Neighborhoods and communities should encourage migrant seniors to engage in community activities to reduce the detrimental impact of the decline in intergenerational emotional support from children to older parents. In addition, migrant seniors can also communicate with each other, so they can know more about the values and thoughts of their children and reduce the generation difference, which can increase migrants' emotional support to their accompanying parents in China.

Some limitations still exist in this study. First, since 58.9% responses of health score are not from migrant seniors themselves but from their children or other people, there may be an agent response bias problem (Rapley, 2003). Given that migrant seniors who report that they are "unhealthy" or they "cannot take care of themselves" only account for 12.4%, it is possible that the health of migrant seniors is slightly overestimated in this study. Second, although the multilevel model is used and yields more precise estimations, the province level rather than neighborhood or community level is used as the level-2. Sometimes a large geographic unit, such as state or province, is far away from individuals and cannot accurately capture their daily social interactions related to health. Therefore, further works are needed in future studies.

References

Bosma, H., Appels, A., Sturmans, F., Grabauskas, V., & Gostautas, A. (1995). Educational level of spouses and risk of mortality: The WHO Kaunas-Rotterdam Intervention Study (KRIS). *International Journal of Epidemiology, 24*(1), 119–126.

Cao, Z., Durden, E., & Mark, T. L. (2009). Comparison of propensity score matching and use of inverse probability of treatment weights. *Value in Health, 12*(3), A26–A26.

Chen, A. (2011). Household income and parent's education: Which is more important for child health? *Journal of Applied Statistics and Management, 30*(6), 960–966.

Cheng, L., Zhang, Y., & Shen, K. (2015). Understanding the pathways of the education-health gradient: Evidence from the Chinese elderly. *China Economic Quarterly, 14*(1), 305–330.

Cui, W. (2003). *Economic analysis on education*. Beijing: Economic Science Press.

Damon, C., & Healther, R. (2013). The effect of education on adult mortality and health: Evidence from Britain. *American Economic Review, 103*(6), 2087–2120.

Ding, Z., You, Q., & Wei, H. (2017). Who is more willing to give economic support for the elderly parents? *China Agricultural University Journal of Social Sciences Edition, 34*(2), 102–111.

Fan, Y. (2016). *The motivations of intergenerational transfers in China: An empirical analysis using CHARLS data.* (Master Degree), Shandong University.

Fei, X. (2013). *Rural China*. Beijing: Zhonghua Book Company.

Grossman, M. (1972). On the concept of health capital and the demand for health. *Journal of Political Economy, 80*(2), 223–255.

Hong, G. (2015). *Causality in a social world: Moderation, meditation and spill-over*. Chichester: John Wiley & Sons Ltd.

Hu, A. (2015). *Theoretical foundation of causal inference in the social sciences*. Beijing: Social Sciences Academic Press.

Hu, A. (2017). Diversity of children's support for their parents in the context of aging: Ideas and behavior. *Social Sciences in China* (3), 77–95.

Jaffe, D. H., Eisenbach, Z., Neumark, Y. D., & Manor, O. (2006). Effects of husbands' and wives' education on each other's mortality. *Social Science and Medicine, 62*(8), 2014–2023.

Jiang, N. (2019). Adult children's education and later-life health of parents in China: The intergenerational effects of human capital investment. *Social Indicators Research, 145,* 257–278.
Li, L. (2004). *Social Medicine*. Beijing: People's Medical Publishing House.
Mak, B., Woo, J., Bowling, A., Wong, F., & Chau, P. H. (2011). Health care prioritization in aging societies: Influence of age, education, health literacy and culture. *Health Policy, 100*(2), 219–233.
Miguel, E., & Kremer, M. (2004). Worms: Identifying impacts on education and health in the presence of treatment externalities. *Econometrica, 72*(1), 159–217.
Monden, C., Lenthe, F. v., Graaf, N. D. D., & Kraaykamp, G. (2003). Partner's and own education: Does who you live with matter for self-assessed health, smoking and excessive alcohol consumption? *Social Science & Medicine, 57*(10), 1901–1912.
Mu, G. (2004). An analysis of the mental support for the elderly. *Journal of Renmin University of China, 18*(4), 124–129.
National Bureau of Statistics. (2018). *Statistical bulletin of national economy and social development in the People's Republic of China in 2017*. Beijing: China Statistics Press.
Nie, H., Pan, Y., Sun, W., & Bao, Y. (2017). Situation of self-perceived health among old floating population in Shanghai: Based on 2015 national family planning dynamic monitoring of the floating population health survey. *Journal of Shanghai Jiao Tong University (Medical Science), 37*(1), 98–101.
Rapley, M. (2003). *Quality of life research: A critical introduction*. United States: Sage Publications Inc.
Ross, C. E., & Wu, C.-L. (1995). The links between education and health. *American Sociological Review, 60*(5), 719–745.
Schnittker, J. (2004). Education and the changing shape of the income gradient in health. *Journal of Health and Social Behavior, 45*(9), 286–305.
Sheng, X., & Tian, Y. (2015). *A sociological research on the medical security of floating population*. Beijing: Social Sciences Academic Press.
Vernon, S. W., & Buffler, P. A. (1988). The status of status inconsistency. *Epidemiologic Reviews, 10*(1), 65–68.
Vettore, M. V., & Aqeeli, A. (2016). The roles of contextual and individual social determinants of oral health-related quality of life in Brazilian adults. *Quality of Life Research, 25*(4), 1029–1042.
Wang, F., & Shi, Y. (2014). Family background, education expectation and college degree attainment: An empirical study based on Shanghai survey. *Chinese Journal of Sociology, 34*(1), 175–195.
Wang, J., Xie, H., & Jiang, B. (2008). *Multilevel Methods and Application*. Beijing: Higher Education Press.
Willis, R. J. (1982). The direction of intergenerational transfers and demographic transition: The Caldwell hypothesis reexamined. *Population and Development Review, 8,* 207–234.
Wu, W. (2009). *Does education cause better health? Explaining educational-related inequalities in health.* (Master Degree), Zhejiang University.
Yamashita, T., & Brown, J. S. (2017). Does cohort matter in the association between education, health literacy and health in the USA? *Health Promotion International, 32*(1), 16–24.
Yuan, F. (2010). *Introduction to pedagogy*. Jinan: Jinan University Press.
Zhang, S., Zhao, Y., Park, A., & Song, X. (2005). Economic returns to schooling in urban China, 1988 to 2001. *Journal of Comparative Economics, 33*(4), 730–752.
Zhang, W., & Li, S. (2004a). Effects of inter-generation support on physical and psychological health status of the oldest-old. *Chinese Journal of Population Science*(S1), 37–42.
Zhang, W., & Li, S. (2004b). Study on the family intergenerational support among the elderly in rural area: Using exponential mixture model to confirm cooperative group theory. *Statistical Research, 21*(5), 33–37.
Zheng, H., Yang, Y., & Land, K. C. (2011). Variance function regression in hierarchical age-period-cohort models: Applications to the study of self-rated health. *American Sociological Review, 76*(6), 955–983.
Zhou, X. (2017). *Chinese feeling: Globalization, social transformation and change of Chinese social mentality*. Beijing: Social Sciences Academic Press.

Kolibri 360 GmbH
Ferdinand-Jühlke-Straße 7
99095 Erfurt, Deutschland
produktsicherheit@kolibri360.de